内秀

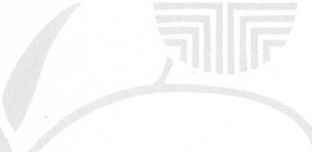

INNER

LOOKING, FEELING AND BEING YOUR B

Also by Xiaolan Zhao, CMD
*Reflections of the Moon on Water: Healing
Women's Bodies and Minds through
Traditional Chinese Wisdom*

BEAUTY

THROUGH TRADITIONAL CHINESE HEALING

XIAOLAN ZHAO, CMD

with

PAULINE COUTURE

Random House Canada

Published by Random House Canada

Copyright © 2011 Xiaolan Zhao

WWW.RANDOMHOUSE.CA

Library and Archives Canada Cataloguing in Publication

Zhao, Xiaolan
Inner beauty : looking, feeling and being your best through traditional Chinese healing / Xiaolan Zhao.

Includes bibliographical references and index.
Issued also in an electronic format.

ISBN 978-0-307-35880-6

1. Beauty, Personal. 2. Women—Health and hygiene. 3. Medicine, Chinese.
4. Alternative medicine. I. Title.

RA778.Z528 2011   646.7'042   C2010-904236-0

Design by Terri Nimmo

Printed in the United States of America

2   4   6   8   9   7   5   3

To all my colleagues at Xiaolan Health Centre,
whose care helps our patients glow
with inner health and beauty

Contents

FOREWORD

Collaborating with Dr. Xiaolan Zhao and becoming her friend and patient has been a journey of learning and opening horizons, in more ways than one.

It took me twelve years of post-secondary education and experience to become a dermatologist and a scientist. Armed with this background, I am able to help hundreds of people every week: workers with occupational skin diseases, teenagers with severe acne, women concerned with protecting their aging skin, students eager to become the next generation of doctors.

And yet I am also keenly aware of the many things for which Western biomedicine does not yet have satisfactory answers; the limitations of treating patients through the narrow lens of a specific specialty rather than as whole beings; and the difficulty in really knowing what patients are experiencing in the short windows of time I have to spend with them.

My colleague Dr. Xiaolan Zhao is an admirable physician and a gifted healer. As an abdominal surgeon in China and a university researcher in Canada, she shares a connection with me to the body of Western medical knowledge. But she is also a highly qualified practitioner of Traditional Chinese Medicine, about which I knew very little until I met her. She tells the story early in this book of how I became her patient. We have also become friends and co-conspirators, enjoying each other's company at work and at play.

Not only has Xiaolan helped me personally, but she has opened my eyes to the depth and breadth of knowledge that TCM has to offer. While my inner scientist continues to want peer-reviewed evidence, my own experience and observation of Xiaolan's practice tell me that thousands of years of traditional knowledge have much to offer that is of great value. I have come to believe that it should be a priority of Western medicine to devote some of its resources to better understanding why TCM analysis and solutions often work as well as, or even better than, the remedies we can offer our patients.

Better still, I think that Xiaolan's ambition of joining hands, East to West, which she has begun to do in her beautiful new wellness centre in midtown Toronto, holds the key to better outcomes for many patients. We have begun to treat some patients together—so far, with excellent results. I have come to feel that there is much promise in this collaboration.

For example: during my twelve years of training and education, I can remember only about six hours of nutrition courses. Now that I have spent more time thinking about the various factors that influence wellness and disease, it seems obvious to me that what we put into our bodies and how we live are crucial determinants of health. Until I got to know Xiaolan, it would never have occurred to me that the condition and beauty of the skin could be linked to the quality of a person's breathing, as this book explains in a whole chapter on breathing—a subject that we take entirely for granted.

And while no Western dermatology manual tells me to do this, I now tell acne and psoriasis patients to avoid spicy foods—because TCM is consistently adamant about this. I have seen Xiaolan's remarkable results with patients who suffer from these and other conditions.

TCM views every patient individually; each treatment is designed for the person, not only for the condition, based on thousands of years of empirical knowledge. Western medicine takes a completely different approach, treating conditions rather than individuals, based on rigorous scientific evidence that can be replicated over and over again. Both approaches have their merits but it can be difficult to reconcile them, and many physicians never attempt to do so.

This book contains many stories from Xiaolan's life and her patients, as well as the patients we have begun to treat together. It also contains much practical information about skin conditions, Xiaolan's treatment approaches and detailed herbal remedies, as well as elements of dialogue between us where we believe there is potential for collaboration between TCM and Western medicine and where we diverge.

This book is intended primarily for an audience of lay people, and it is mostly written in direct language, often using non-medical terms. Despite this, I think that my Western colleagues will find it interesting and revealing. I hope that they, as I have, will welcome this journey of discovery into what Xiaolan's world and our patients have to teach us.

Sandy Skotnicki, M.D.

INTRODUCTION

I am delighted to write an introduction to this book.

I met Dr. Xiaolan Zhao in 1990. At that time, she had just started her Traditional Chinese Medicine practice in Canada. She had received her MD degree in China in 1977 and her Doctor of Traditional Chinese Medicine degree in China in 1985.

Dr. Xiaolan Zhao is an expert in 正骨 (zhèng gǔ). "Zhèng" means *adjust*; "gǔ" means *bones*. Zhèng gǔ is a 5,000-year-old ancient Chinese treasure. There are very few doctors who excel at zhèng gǔ.

After meeting Dr. Zhao, I introduced one of my friends to her who had a dislocated elbow joint. Dr. Zhao applied her zhèng gǔ techniques, and within seconds, she corrected my friend's dislocated elbow. That power has been left in my heart forever.

Dr. Zhao is a very successful expert in Traditional Chinese Medicine. She has used her expertise to treat thousands of difficult cases from all over the world, with remarkable healing results. Many MDs and other medical professionals see her for acupuncture, Chinese herbs, and tuī ná (Chinese massage).

I have read her excellent first book, *Reflections of the Moon on Water*, in which Dr. Zhao shares the essence of 5,000 years of Traditional Chinese Medicine, especially the essence of *The Yellow Emperor's Canon*, which is the authority book of

Traditional Chinese Medicine. Her new book, *Inner Beauty*, offers great guidance to help women gain wisdom and knowledge in the use of herbs and also offers practices to prevent and heal female challenges.

A human being has body, mind and spirit. Spirit is soul. Every system, every organ and every cell has a soul. Soul is the "boss" of a human being, and of every system, organ and cell. Modern medicine focuses on Jing, which is matter. Traditional Chinese medicine focuses on Qi, which is vital energy or life force—and it is Qi that *Inner Beauty* is most concerned with.

So many people are preoccupied with making themselves beautiful. They invest huge amounts of effort and money to improve their appearance. Dr. Zhao brings great wisdom to the public: *in order to have outer beauty, you must first have inner beauty.* Inner beauty will bring outer beauty if you balance your Yin and Yang and your Five Elements, which are wood, fire, earth, metal and water.

In Traditional Chinese Medicine, wood represents the Liver, Gallbladder, eyes and tendons, and anger in the emotional body. The fire element represents the Heart, Small Intestine, tongue and blood vessels, and depression and anxiety in the emotional body. The earth element represents the Spleen, Stomach, mouth, muscles, lips and gums, and worry in the emotional body. The metal element includes the Lungs, Large Intestine, nose and skin, and grief and sadness in the emotional body. The water element represents the Kidneys, Urinary Bladder, ears and bones, and fear in the emotional body. To have inner beauty is to balance the Five Elements and their corresponding Organs, tissues, and cells.

I highly recommend Dr. Xiaolan Zhao's book, *Inner Beauty*, to everyone. Learn the wisdom and practical techniques shared in this book to find your inner beauty, and your outer beauty will follow.

I wish you will receive great benefits from the teaching and practices of this book.

I am happy and honoured to share these words.

Wishing you good health and happiness,

Dr. and Master Zhìgāng Shā 志鋼沙

Founder, Institute of Soul Healing and Enlightenment

AUTHOR'S
INTRODUCTION

"Xiaolan, I'm in so much pain . . . please see me right away, it feels like a knife in my leg!" This cry of help from one of my long-time patients came in an urgent phone call; my heart sank. I knew that she must have—against my advice—undergone yet another round of cosmetic surgery.

Francine is a beautiful, vibrant woman in her mid-fifties. She has everything she could ever want—except for a flat abdomen and skinny thighs. For years she has been obsessed with sculpting her body to look more like a magazine model—Western society's ideal of external beauty.

This time, she had taken a bigger risk than ever before: a third liposuction on her thighs, abdomen and back. Francine told me that she was taking the anti-inflammatory drugs and antibiotics that her surgeon had prescribed, and she was popping painkillers like candy, but they weren't helping. The pain was constant and overwhelming. I asked her if she had been to Emergency, but she begged me to see her right away. "Please, Xiaolan, I trust you. It's you I want to see."

I agreed to see her over my lunch hour. When I saw her anxious husband and adult son and daughter carrying her into the clinic, I realized that the situation was serious. She was shaking, in so much pain that she could not even stand. Between sobs, Francine's daughter told me she had never seen her strong, loving mother in such a state. All three pleaded with me to do something for her; Francine's husband looked stricken. I examined her quickly, but I knew instantly what was happening. Her left calf was swollen, hard as a rock, and hot to the touch, while her hands were in a cold sweat. "Francine," I said, "you need an ultrasound right away. I think you have a blood clot in your ankle. But you're really lucky—so far, it's not in your heart or your brain."

Francine went to her surgeon for the ultrasound and it confirmed my diagnosis. I prescribed Chinese herbs, rest and elevation of her legs at home, while her surgeon put her on blood thinners—for life.

Francine survived the blood clot, and for the moment she does have skinny thighs. But is she any happier than before?

This story is not unique in my practice. Many of my patients undergo surgeries and procedures that I believe are harmful and unnecessary—all in the name of "beauty."

Over the years, I have treated thousands of patients, and I see true beauty in all of them. But I have come to realize that many of these women do not see themselves as beautiful. They suffer terribly because they long to meet standards of beauty that are artificial, temporary or non-existent. Magazine images are manipulated with airbrushing and computer software. The "perfect beauty" in ads does not exist.

It is hard to overestimate the damage that this societal standard does to the self-esteem of young girls and women who see that media imagery of the ideal woman is so far from their own reality and that they can never meet these expectations. The aspects of their beings that truly matter: their goodness, their intelligence, their radiant good health—seem to pale in significance beside these mirages.

Indulging in obsession over superficial beauty is not the Chinese way. Having been raised in the Eastern philosophy, it took me some time to realize how debilitating this situation can be. I decided that I wanted to write a book that would explain that the only true beauty is that which comes from within, and that it starts from a healthy and balanced life.

In Traditional Chinese Medicine (TCM), we speak of the Three Treasures, which define life and health: Jing (精), Qi (氣) and Shen (神). My first book, *Reflections of the Moon on Water,* dealt extensively with the first of the Three Treasures, Jing (精), or Essence. It introduced readers to the basic elements of TCM: Yin and Yang, the Five Elements, the Zang-Fu Organs, and the holistic, causal, preventive and natural approaches it offers to maintaining balance and lifelong health. Taking care of our bodies and ensuring that we have what we need to keep ourselves healthy and balanced leads to energy, optimism and the ability to undertake the activities we choose for ourselves. When we do not take care of ourselves, all Three Treasures weaken and our bodies become imbalanced.

This book, although it briefly covers the basics of TCM, deals primarily with Qi (氣), the second of the Three Treasures, the life force itself. The traditional character for Qi, 氣, evokes the steam rising from cooking rice and its transformative character, in both the material (rice) and the immaterial (steam) states. The Qi that rises and descends in our bodies is both inherited in our genetic blueprint and created every day through our diet, breathing and activities. Qi travels through the fourteen Meridians of the body, from inside to outside, from side to side and from top to toe. The state of our Qi manifests directly and openly in the skin, our largest organ and the map of our experiences and state of health.

When women undergo invasive cosmetic surgeries, they are tampering with their bodies' amazing systems for balance and self-healing. The connective tissues and Meridians are damaged, blocked and broken. The body's capacity to recover from stress and injury is diminished, and patients are rarely ever entirely the same afterwards. The best I can do is to offer TCM techniques to help lessen the trauma.

As a surgeon, I know the risks of any kind of surgery. While these cosmetic procedures may give patients a temporary high, my view is that it is impossible to be happy if you do not accept who you are. Most of these patients subsequently experience a great letdown when they realize that the surgery has not changed them beyond the superficial, and that the results do not last.

The idea of beauty has inspired some of humanity's most luminous poetry and songs, images and books. We all want to be beautiful. But the truth is, our external body is always in transition, impermanent. We cannot stop or slow down the inexorable process of aging that each of us is undergoing every day. The pursuit of the impermanent external forms of beauty leads inevitably to suffering.

On the other hand, the pursuit of inner beauty, health and balance is endlessly rewarding. This book is not a conventional "beauty" book, and you will find no makeup and fashion tips here. What you *will* find is a philosophical and practical approach to being your best and healthiest self, so that you radiate with the vibrant Qi that courses through your body and projects your inner beauty.

At my Toronto wellness clinic, Xiaolan Health Centre, I have sought to bring together the knowledge and wisdom of both Eastern and Western medicine to provide effective health care that balances all the unique concerns and dimensions of each person's life. Whether we target a specific affliction, such as chronic pain, or concentrate on being more proactive about long-term wellness, we strive to provide that necessary balance— in the subtle interplay between nutrition and emotion, fitness and self-awareness, body and spirit.

It is my mission to find ways to bring together two great medical traditions to complement, support and learn from one another. The East offers us pathways to understanding and treatment that have stood the test of five thousand years. It's a tradition that believes in treating the whole person, not isolated symptoms, because it sees symptoms simply as signs, as a language by which the body expresses its need to be whole again.

From the West, on the other hand, we take proven approaches to diagnosis and care and weave them together with the best of alternative therapies. We appreciate that there are insights to be gained from science, that technologies can help reveal problems and repair what is damaged—but again, never in isolation, only as part of an overall assessment of how patients are living their lives. Above all, we focus not just on treatment but, far more importantly, on prevention. We want to help patients take control of their personal health, to begin a journey toward living a fuller, happier life. In doing so we hope to make Xiaolan Health Centre both a welcome alternative and an inspiring model for a humane, holistic, multi-faceted approach to wellness—a place where patients can find balance.

After my first book was published, I found that many people asked me for more information about practical ways to use TCM principles and Chinese herbs in their own lives and self-care. I decided that my next book would contain a significant reference section to help readers understand how TCM solutions can help them manage various conditions, particularly those related to the skin.

What's more, the reference section—found in the middle of this book—attempts to take advantage of both Eastern and Western medical traditions. With the help of my colleague Dr. Sandy Skotnicki, a respected dermatologist, I have explored how both traditions can work together to provide patients with the best care and optimal healing. Throughout the reference section, Sandy has commented on how Western medicine addresses these conditions, and on occasion she and I have entered into a dialogue about the best approaches.

The rest of the book explores the many aspects of inner beauty that I see every day in my patients. Through anecdotes and case studies, I invite you to think about your ideas of beauty, the body and the spirit in different ways through different stages of life and health conditions that you may encounter. In this book, I have concentrated largely on the skin, which faithfully projects what is going on in your body, mind and spirit. The teachings and practice of TCM are inclusive, welcoming and inspirational. It is my most heartfelt wish that this book may help you achieve inner peace and the beauty that radiates from it.

CHAPTER ONE

WHAT IS BEAUTY?

内秀 *(Nèi Xiù)*

One day, when I was four years old, my grandmother brought me to her workplace—a factory that was making traditional Chinese painted wooden suitcases. This must have been during the school holidays, because many of the factory's employees had their small children with them at work that day.

I, grandmother's little princess, was perched on a ladder beside her, happily eating my lunch as I "supervised" her work. Next to us, her colleague's six-year-old son was watching jealously. He wanted that ladder, and I was in the way. Sneaking up behind me, he suddenly pushed me hard. In one terrifying moment, my happiness dissolved into terror as my spoon caught my lip and gashed it deeply; it began to bleed profusely.

At that moment, I believed my grandmother must have had three hands: in the very instant that she grabbed me to staunch the bleeding, she stopped her colleague from beating her son and enfolded the little miscreant in her free arm. "Don't punish him. He didn't mean to hurt her. Can't you see how afraid he is? Don't worry, little man, the doctor will be able to help Xiaolan." I began to howl even more loudly. She should have been protecting me and punishing him, not comforting him! The outrage was worse than the pain!

When we returned from the hospital, where they had repaired my lip (five stitches!), the little boy and his mother were waiting for us. The mother had brought congee (rice porridge), knowing that I would not be able to eat solid food with my injured mouth. The little boy apologized with real sincerity, and he was always my friend after that.

My grandmother's compassion and forgiveness changed that boy, and me along with him. She lived in the moment, and always saw the opportunity in mistakes. Sometimes I run my tongue over the little bump that has remained on my lower lip all my life and earned me the nickname "little meat lip" from my sisters. It always reminds me of the inner beauty and wisdom that shone in my grandmother's face, and I am sure that her spirit is with me.

> Happy people never count hours as they pass.
> —*Chinese proverb*

ACCEPTANCE

As a small child, I thought my grandmother was the most beautiful woman on earth; this has shaped my idea of beauty all my life. She gave me unconditional love and acceptance, drawing on her vast store of wisdom as she raised me from shortly after birth to the age of six. She cared for me and my three older siblings during this period when the Communist Chinese government had ordered my parents to live elsewhere—my father to work in another city and my mother to do hard labour on a re-education farm.

In this formative period of my early childhood, my grandmother was the only parent I knew. Like parents everywhere, she was determined that my life would be easier than hers had been. She protected me from harm and from the judgment of others—especially children, who can be so cruel—no matter what I did. Although I did not always understand that she was doing this, she always accepted who I was at every stage of my life.

I feel her presence every day. Remembering her "being" is deeply moving to me—especially in light of her own early child-hood of intense suffering. You see, my grandmother was one of the last wave of little Chinese girls to endure the horrors of bound feet. In 1908, when she was three years old, she was sub-jected to the systematic breaking and putrefaction of the soft bones and flesh of her feet in order to turn them into three-inch "golden lotuses"—the standard of beauty for upper-class women.

As a result, for the rest of her life, she could walk only in great pain. The sad irony that foot-binding was outlawed in 1912, just four years later, meant that she would be marked in the eyes of the Communist regime as one of those who should be forced to work even harder because of their suspect origins. The women who lived through these times learned tremendous discipline and devotion to their families and to each other, channelling their suffering into love and selfless support for others.

On my parents' return from their time away from us, they were horrified to find that I, their youngest child whom they barely knew, had become "wild grass"—fearless, free and happy. In those difficult and repressive times, they were afraid I might do something that could place me—and possibly my entire family—in danger. I had no such sense of imminent danger, since my grandmother had sheltered me completely from harm and allowed me to develop freely under her protective wing.

Hatred corrodes the vessel in which it is stored.
—*Chinese proverb*

My grandmother's life was one of great hardship in many ways. And yet she found beauty in every moment. She accepted her life as it was; she did not fight its reality, dwell in the past or project into the future. She was intensely present and conscious of the universe and her place in it. On market days around the

full moon, she would practise the old Buddhist custom of awareness and compassion, buying fish, eels or birds to release into
the wild to give thanks. She believed that each of these animals
had its own spirit, which was at one with humans and the universe as a whole. At the full moon and the new moon, her diet
was vegetarian for three days. Every day, she burned incense and
prayed for the health of the whole family. She was unburdened
with anger and bitterness from the past.

To me, my grandmother was the living embodiment of the
Chinese characters you see at the beginning of this chapter,
which mean both "inner beauty" and "inner wisdom." Although
nothing I have experienced in my life can compare to foot-
binding, I am filled with admiration and gratitude for my
grandmother's love and her acceptance of the family's destiny,
which prepared me for the challenges I would face.

Today in my practice, I encourage my patients to achieve this
state of acceptance, from which a peaceful and balanced life
flows. I find that those who are able to move in this direction
inevitably heal more quickly than others. Alice, a diminutive
woman of Russian origin, is one such patient. She has shown
great courage and acceptance.

Alice had lived for a number of years with vitiligo, an autoimmune disease that destroys skin pigmentation in spreading
patches. I asked her how she had managed to accept her condition so gracefully. She told me that she had learned the concept
of acceptance through something that had happened many years
previously. Alice and her husband had emerged from a children's
hospital with their nine-year-old son, freshly diagnosed with
insulin-dependent diabetes. Her husband was very upset at this
news. He was thinking of the rest of his son's life—first under
the constant parental monitoring of his insulin levels and injec-
tions, and then, later on, under the restrictions this might impose
on his future, as he would have to take over his own care.

As they were leaving the hospital and experiencing this intense emotion, they ran into a friend. When they told her their news, she said, "You are so fortunate! Your son will be able to manage his diabetes and live a normal life. But our neighbour's son is dying of cancer, and there is nothing to be done."

Alice and her husband immediately realized that their friend was right. They accepted their diabetic son's condition and moved on, ensuring that he had a normal, active and happy life. Through their example, their son also accepted his condition and learned to manage it cheerfully and competently. Their son's doctor even asked Alice to speak to another Russian-speaking mother who was having great difficulty accepting her daughter's diabetes.

This experience made it much easier, when the time came, for Alice to accept her vitiligo as a simple cosmetic problem without real consequences. As her skin lost its pigmentation, it became as soft and smooth as a baby's, and its patchiness dissolved into one creamy colour. Unlike other patients who do not accept their disease and fight it by going to tanning salons or submitting to cosmetic procedures, Alice suffered no depression or pain. Her husband gave her unwavering support; he called her "Honey Leopard" and told her every day that he loved her and found her beautiful, supporting her healing process as much as he could.

IMPERMANENCE

Late one night a few years ago, the phone rang and woke me. Rarely does a late-night call bring good news: when my sister gently broke the news that my grandmother had died, I immediately felt a great sense of loss. Never again would her luminous eyes meet mine or her kind smile reassure me that all was well; never again would I be able to snuggle into her comforting warmth and listen to the endless stories that I loved so much, or caress her lined face and laugh with her.

"What happened?" I sobbed. "Was she ill? Did she suffer?"

In her calm voice, my sister assured me that our grandmother had not suffered. On the contrary, she had prepared and served a joyous Friday dinner with the family and gone to bed serene and happy. The next morning, she had risen early, bathed herself and changed into brand-new clothes. Then she had gone to bed and never woken up. The cleaning lady had found her, peaceful and beautiful as ever, the incense still burning on the table beside her bed. My sister comforted me: "Grandmother has returned to her original home." Through my tears, I began to feel calmer too. I knew my sister was right.

My grandmother's earthly form has dissolved, but her inner beauty lives on in me and in everyone who knew her. Her essence is forever. In contrast to the beauty that emanated from every atom of my grandmother's being, external beauty is truly impermanent. One of my long-time patients, Laurie, told me a story that brings this home. At her high school reunion, everyone there recognized her, but she recognized almost no one. She was shocked that the girl who had been the most beautiful, the most popular and the most successful in her high school days—the queen of the prom—was almost impossible to recognize. The gorgeous blonde Laurie remembered was a tired, middle-aged mother of three, drinking rye whisky from a flask in the bathroom. She had never had a career, and she was deeply disillusioned with her high school sweetheart, now a long-inattentive husband.

Laurie had been a tomboy, an outsider. She remembered how her Italian working-class father, worried that his daughter, with her fierce independence and unconventional looks, would never find a husband, had always said to her, "Laurie, it's a good thing you're so smart." At the time, she had not thought much about it. But as she looked at the disillusioned beauty queen, it dawned on her that she had coasted on her early successes, based on her looks. During that time, Laurie had focused on her inner purpose, living a life of authenticity, rooted in the present moment. This had served her well. Because her inner purpose and her external life were so closely aligned, she was successful on her own terms, both professionally and personally. She felt only compassion for her former schoolmate.

THE TRICKERY OF TIME

Shortly after my grandmother's far-away death, an elderly patient of mine came to me with a fluffy orange bundle. She told me that the little chow puppy was a gift that she believed I needed. I took the squirming puppy in my arms. As I looked into his eyes, I immediately felt that he was somehow the embodiment of my grandmother's spirit: "She is here, in this moment!" I thought.

Nangua is pumpkin-coloured. But the reason I gave him this Mandarin name (*Nangua* means "pumpkin") also has to do with the image of the pumpkin in Chinese folklore: a humble, sturdy, healthy vegetable without intellectual pretensions. We humans are the ones with intellectual pretensions. Alone in the animal kingdom, we are psychologically affected by the idea of aging and the passage of time. Nangua does not share my anxiety about the day, someday soon, when he will no longer be with me.* And if he could understand—as I sometimes feel he does—he would think I am very silly to worry about this.

Seventeen is a very old age for a dog—even for a super-healthy dog like Nangua, on whom I lavish not only affection but daily herbs and vitamins, and occasional preventive acupuncture. Every morning, Nangua awakes happy and ready to walk with me to work. He is totally absorbed by whatever delights present themselves: an interesting plant, a nice pole or tree on which to relieve himself, a laughing child or a squirrel

---

* Sadly, Nangua died shortly after this book was finished.

worth chasing. He shares this happiness with me and reminds me how much there is to enjoy in the world.

At night, if all is safe and quiet and I am well, he sleeps when I sleep. But if there is danger, or if I am not feeling well, Nangua stands guard and protects me. He is never concerned with something that happened last week or something that might happen next year. Every day is a new, beautiful day. Every walk is a happy walk. Every sleep is a good sleep. Nangua is a good teacher; he reminds me that it is futile to wish for my grandmother's earthly presence—and yet, that she is always with me. He reminds me of the joy that we can find in being, rather than doing.

Unfortunately, doing is valued much more highly than being in Western societies. In most Eastern societies, older people are revered for their wisdom and experience. They are included, consulted and pampered—and therefore, they are less fearful of the aging process and the passage of time. The concept of time is fundamentally different between Eastern and Western cultures, and is reflected in the languages we speak. In my mother tongue, Mandarin, there is neither past nor future tense. All verbs are present tense—and this encourages the concept of an ongoing now, the value of being versus doing.

In Western societies, it is common to hear the expression "Time is money." If you are not productive and doing something, you are not valued. Time spent taking care of your health is not built into many people's schedules. This leads to decisions that can have devastating effects on your health and your life, such as eating a diet of greasy fast food, or making quick decisions, uninformed by wisdom and compassion. While the depreciation of aging and wisdom is harmful to everyone, it is most devastating for women, who feel they must conform to a standard that is entirely unrealistic and often find themselves cast aside while they still have so much to give.

Maria, a sophisticated and accomplished professional in the media world, has begun to lie about her age or refuse to give it. Why? Because despite the shelf full of awards she has received for her work, she fears that putting a number on the passage of time in her life will depreciate her market value and actually threaten her ability to make a living.

She says that in her male-dominated sector, "I know that it will be a liability; it's the truth, you can't do anything about it. No one is going to say you're too old, they're just not going to call. I think about getting something done for that reason, even though I can't afford it."

You can imagine how much suffering this entails.

IDENTIFICATION

There is a French saying: "Il faut souffrir pour être belle" (one must suffer to be beautiful), and certainly this proverb reminds me of the old Chinese practice of foot-binding. Whenever I see advertising for extremely high-heeled shoes, I am reminded that this noxious attitude permeates many cultures. So many women are in thrall to the idea that they must impose costly and toxic practices on their bodies in order to meet whatever social norms of beauty are of their time. Almost all the girls who wear six-inch heels today will suffer from arthritis and joint pain in their backs, hips, knees and ankles for many years. For some women, the price is even higher, simply because they are so desperate to improve their appearance, to attract a man or to try to escape their natural and inevitable aging process. Why would anyone risk dying prematurely and leaving behind their loved ones for such a reason?

A good friend of mine told me the story of one of her clients, a driven, ambitious woman who died after seven hours on the operating table while undergoing a facelift, liposuction and several other cosmetic procedures—all at once. The woman was attractive, healthy and accomplished, but this was never enough for her. She was always rushing, always busy. Her time was precious because she always had more meetings to run, more money to earn and more awards to win. She was a perfectionist in all things, and she placed these same kinds of demands on her body as she approached middle age.

She did not even want to take the time to let her body recover from each of these traumatic interventions one at a time. Like many powerful, wealthy people, she had a great capacity for persuasion, and she was able to convince her doctor to perform these extremely risky procedures despite his misgivings—and despite the objections of her distraught husband.

I see many cases like this, of women constantly wanting more and being in denial about the natural aging process. Fortunately, it remains rare that they pay the ultimate price of life itself, as this woman did. But so many women I see simply cannot accept the changes in their body as they age.

For all of us, identity is so wrapped up in our external appearance that it is easy to lose our way. When this happens, we do not always reflect on the consequences of the desperate actions many women take to maintain their youthful looks. The suffering that I see around me is often caused by an inability to appreciate and honour who we are. What we do is not who we are. What we look like is not who we are. We are not our intelligence quotient, our physical dimensions or our gifts, however marvellous they may be. So why do we become disconnected from who we are and unable to live in harmony with what is?

Sometimes this happens because people come to identify with something other than who they truly are, such as the appearance of their bodies and faces at a fleeting moment in time. They may fixate on the future and become obsessed with their career ambitions or money. Or they may be born and raised in situations where they identify totally with a religion, a nationality or historical conflicts—anything that allows them to think that they are superior and apart from other humans and the environment, or that they are victims. People are constantly judging themselves rather than living their lives in the moment. This false identification is not rooted in consciousness, which places us squarely in the universe as an integral part of it, living the moments of our lives as they unfold, and discovering the inner beauty in ourselves and in others.

Sometimes it takes a crisis to change this. One of my patients completely transformed her life as the result of a sudden change in her health that forced her to let go of her identification with her external beauty. As a pretty and sociable young woman, Susan had "peaches and cream" skin. She was popular with her circle of friends and often went to parties and dances, in part to distract herself from her dysfunctional family. At eighteen, her inner sadness suddenly caught up with her and surfaced in her skin.

In the space of a few days, she went from a nonchalant existence in which she relied heavily on her looks to a painful condition of severe acne and self-consciousness. Her face was suddenly covered with bleeding scabs and sores. She no longer felt able to go out and expose herself to the people she had thought of as friends to that point.

For a description of acne at different stages of life, and recipes for both topical and internal herbal remedies, see pages 79 to 88.

SURRENDER

Over the next eight or nine years, Susan embarked on a spiritual journey of inner and outer healing that eventually led her to my clinic. Like many of my patients, she told me that I was the last resort. By then, Susan was severely depressed. Her face was covered with acne—red, angry spots, swollen and full of pus. She had stomach pains, bloating and constipation. I looked her in the eye and told her, "In three months, your skin will be like mine—as long as we are working together."

She said, "I trust you; I will follow your advice." From that moment on, she took her herbs and vitamins; she continued with psychotherapy; she began to practise meditation and conscious breathing exercises daily; and she came for regular TCM treatments, all of which helped her to release her emotions. Our experience together was the culmination of Susan's long journey. Once she had learned to accept her imperfect family and surrender to "what is," her skin began to heal.

Within three months, she had regained both smooth skin and the self-confidence to make major changes in her life—but she did not return to the life she had led before. Her experience had transformed her and led her to a different path. Susan went back to school and has now embarked on a career that she loves, sharing her journey to help other people.

The concept of surrender is a difficult one to understand. It sounds like defeat, yet is anything but. In the East, to surrender means to yield to the forces in your life and to work with them rather than wasting energy fighting what is. When we stop resisting what is actually happening in our lives in that moment, we gain the space to do what we need to do, which may involve profound change. But as long as we are busily opposing these life forces, we cannot even see what needs to be done. In TCM, this yielding, enveloping power is the great source of feminine energy—Yin, which we will discuss in Chapter Two.

Sandy came into my clinic on the recommendation of a friend. Her life was extremely full at the best of times: she was a "hockey mom" to three delightful young boys, a busy dermatologist with a prestigious downtown clinic, an academic with both teaching and heavy research responsibilities, and a wife in a marriage under stress.

I remember seeing her for the first time, a classic North American beauty: tall, perfectly proportioned and slender, with long auburn hair. Sandy was clearly a high-achieving professional with a huge capacity for work and the demands of personal life. She worked hard, increasingly in demand for her expertise, and juggled a demanding and sophisticated downtown dermatology clinic and academic activities with her growing family.

There was just one problem: her capacity to absorb stress had reached the tipping point. Her visibility had been increasing steadily, and she was being asked to do more lectures. Her beloved mother had fallen gravely ill and was dying, and her father was leaning heavily on her for emotional support. All this was taking its toll. Her beautiful hair was shedding. Her lips were chapped and she projected no energy, no spark. She was catching back-to-back colds and couldn't shake them. An incident at one of her sons' hockey games made her realize that she was tired, sick and cranky—just not herself. She needed help.

The good news is that she had the courage to explore new solutions. She came to our clinic with an open heart and an open mind. I knew then and there that we could get along. For the first three weeks, she came every seven days. As any TCM practitioner would, we did not treat her condition in isolation. I looked at Sandy as a whole, the person whose symptoms were flaring up in this way, and I sought to understand what was going on in her body, in her mind and in her spirit. I treated her with herbs, acupuncture, 推拿 tuī ná (Chinese massage aligned with the Meridians) and advice about her lifestyle and diet.

Within three weeks of that initial visit, Sandy's health began to improve, from the inside out: her hair stopped shedding, her cold disappeared and her energy began to return. Slowly, she was able to deal with her difficult situation and let go of the intense emotions that were blocking her energy. Despite the very real problems that she faced, Sandy began to function much more capably and with far less tension in her life.

We talked about her emotions and her stress at home and at work. Sandy became intrigued with the idea that TCM deals with the whole person rather than the person's conditions and symptoms. This confirmed her own experience that the skin of many of her patients was expressing distress at what was going on in their bodies and in their lives. She felt that her patients would benefit from support for their emotional issues as well as their more visible symptoms. Thus Sandy and I began a dialogue about what we could learn from each other.

Having begun my medical career as a Western-trained general surgeon, I have a good understanding of Sandy's philosophical and scientific framework, and I know that it has much to offer. I was enthusiastic about the idea of bridging the divide between East and West in the company of someone who is open to exploring how we can link these valuable pools of knowledge to work together in the best interests of our patients. Many patients are confused and distressed by the distance between these two great traditions—especially when they obtain contradictory advice from their physicians.

For more on stress-related skin conditions, including chapped lips and hair loss, see the reference section, beginning on page 77. The section includes recipes for herbal remedies, both topical and internal.

BEYOND SKIN-DEEP

As Sandy and I began to talk, we also began to explore what beauty means to men and women today. In Sandy's practice, the answer tends to be straightforward: beauty equals youth, and the vast majority of her patients are seeking to reverse the effects of aging, or even forestall them well before they appear. Both Sandy and I see patients who are deeply anxious about their own value in a media-driven culture that places a disproportionate importance on skin-deep beauty.

These destructive messages are hammered home from all quarters in our society: if you look better, you will do better and you will feel better. Unless you have youthful, smooth skin, you won't get a boyfriend or a girlfriend. If you look old, you won't get a job. If you are disfigured by acne or psoriasis, you won't have friends. No wonder so many men and women suffer from low self-esteem.

Sandy has told me that even women in their twenties come to see her, asking for their first Botox treatments. I must admit that I find this very disturbing. My earliest childhood experiences—not only with my beloved grandmother, but throughout Chinese society—taught me to treasure the aging woman as a source of strength, comfort, happiness and delight.

All of us are also very much shaped by our life experiences. Sandy and I share the opinion that despite the value that society places on beauty, it can be hard on the person who projects it to others. If life can be hard for a beautiful woman, it can be even harder for a beautiful, intelligent one.

Some women are so self-conscious about their appearance that they will not leave home to go jogging or grocery shopping without full makeup. I sometimes wonder if their own families know what these women really look like.

Greta, for example, is a brilliant and successful woman with a global network of friends and admirers. She has a loving relationship with her children. But still, she is never satisfied with her appearance. Over the years, she has had facelifts, tummy tucks, liposuction and a breast reduction. These painful procedures have not solved whatever problems Greta thought she had with her appearance. Worse than that, they have actually caused great stress on her general health. She is restless, with agitated sleep. Her stomach is constantly painful and bloated.

She has taken drastic measures to alter her appearance, but she has not changed the habits that brought her to the point of wanting cosmetic surgery in the first place. She continues to overeat and to drink too much. The fat that is sucked out in the surgical procedures soon returns to her midriff, and she is nearing the time when no responsible surgeon will want to repeat the procedure. What will she do then?

Greta can afford to pay for prominent cosmetic doctors. Her operations have not changed her dramatically—yet. But I am concerned that these kinds of transformations take Greta, and other patients, further and further away from the essence of who they really are. It seems to become easier and easier with each intervention to accept changes that are more dramatic over time.

In our clinic, we have treated many women whose faces appear frozen like a mask, who cannot express themselves with their facial muscles, so that people who love them begin to feel sealed off from them. In the worst cases, it is difficult to look at these women because the message that they are sending to the world is one of profound unhappiness in their own skins. Their Qi is totally blocked and no longer flows to their faces.

I perceive these efforts to push back against the aging process as a source of endless suffering. I would love our patients always to see themselves as beautiful. Wrinkles are the map of a life, to be honoured and valued. If you are comfortable with your body, you will also be healthier in every way. While I support the well-being of my patients who choose to undergo cosmetic procedures, I continue to feel strongly that there is another way.

It is certainly possible for a person who is sixty or seventy or eighty years old to appear decades younger at first glance. But this comes at a steep price. It reminds me of an astronaut walking in space, drifting away after losing the link to the mother ship. The loss of contact with who we really are is too high a price to pay for the illusion of youth—an illusion that is based on an ideal that does not truly exist.

DEFINING BEAUTY

Her fingers were like the blades of the young white-grass
Her skin was like congealed ointment
Her neck was like the tree-grub
Her teeth were like melon seeds
Her forehead cicada-like
Her eyebrows like silkworm antennae
What dimples, as she artfully smiled!
How lovely her eyes, with the black and white so well defined!
    Shuo Ren, the 57th poem in THE BOOK OF ODES

No one describing a beautiful woman today would compare her facial features to insect body parts, as the Shuo Ren did in *The Book of Odes*! But there is no one consensus about what beauty is, and there are dramatic shifts in aesthetic appreciation over time.

The period of the Tang Dynasty (618–907) is known for the freedom enjoyed by Chinese women (at least those with some means). Period images portray women full of energy, showing off

> Everything has beauty, but not everyone sees it.
> —CONFUCIUS

their athletic and artistic skills—playing polo on horseback, painting and carving. The Tang emperors viewed plump women as symbols of their own wealth and privilege. Today, the ceramic figures of elegant women of the court that have been found in tombs from the period are sometimes called "fat ladies" because of their fleshy faces.

In the millennium during which upper-class Chinese women had bound feet, it was more common to praise delicacy and slenderness, which may have resulted in part from the weakness and suffering of women unable to walk normally without great pain.

Even today, Western fashion magazines showcase models who are so thin that the look has been called "heroin chic," while in some developing countries (such as Mauritania), young girls are fattened to morbid obesity in order to be considered marriageable. Whatever the demands of a society's canons of beauty, women tend to internalize the devastating message that they are not acceptable as they really are. This always results in suffering.

Many people of all ages do not realize that the tall, slender models who fill the pages of today's fashion magazines do not look at all like their pictures when you meet them in jeans on the street. Their pictures are highly processed and manipulated by computer software that makes legs longer and thinner, eyes and breasts larger, waists and hips smaller and skin smoother. And the problem is global. In Asia, for instance, cosmetic companies make huge profits selling whitening creams, and some young women undergo plastic surgery to make their eyes rounder—all in the name of beauty. I cannot help but agree with my friend the art dealer Jane Corkin that the entire concept of beauty has been "hijacked" to some extent.

When I first came to Canada in 1988, I was untouched by the kind of beauty propaganda that is now so invasively present—and increasingly, not only in the West, but also in the modern China I no longer know very well. I had been raised to believe that what mattered was my intellect, my achievements, my loyalty to my family and friends. My mother had taught me that soft curves were becoming in a woman, and that staying healthy and strong was the priority for my management of my body.

TCM defines beauty through external signs of internal health: radiant Qi, flowing freely and visibly in beautiful skin, hair and teeth, and visible energy.

I was surprised when I first came here to see how much emphasis was placed on slenderness as an essential element of beauty. To my surprise, I found that some of my patients in this country of abundance displayed signs of malnutrition I had not seen since I had left China, because they were starving themselves of essential nutrients in an attempt to lose weight.

Over time, and despite my upbringing, I even found myself giving in to this insidious influence. I began to eat less, perhaps less than I should have. It was not until a friend pointed this out to me that I began to realize how powerful are the media images with which we are surrounded—even those of us who never watch television!—and how vigilant we must be to protect ourselves and to ensure that our inner health and beauty come first.

Although I am saddened by the consequences of these pressures on our patients, I always try to remember my grandmother's way: acceptance and unconditional love. In keeping with her teachings, I do not judge the women I know who decide that they need "work" in the elusive pursuit of ideal beauty.

TCM requires us to take responsibility for our own health and accompanies us in this process. I advise these patients as best I can to support them and their general health throughout the procedures and therapies they choose to undergo. I continue to draw inspiration from TCM's history, in which practitioners were paid as long as patients remained healthy rather than for repairing sick bodies. I do wish there were more incentives for preventive medicine today.

I regret that except for the rare cases where the procedures are correcting a serious deformity or functional problem, mostly I do not feel that these expensive treatments make the women

Beauty gives pleasure to the senses and reaches us at the deepest level of our souls. It can emanate from within or be constructed, as in art, music, literature or architecture. Beauty constructed, comes from the soul of the maker; stretching the minds and stimulating the senses of its audience to arrive at a pleasurable place. Complete beauty is the prescription to enduring calm. Once tasted, it is hard to imagine living without it.

—JANE CORKIN, ART DEALER

I know any happier. Sandy and I sometimes have different perspectives on this issue, and also lively discussions from time to time.

Beauty does not come from endless cosmetic procedures. It does not come from makeup or clothing or money or status. When patients are truly engaged with me during a treatment, nothing else exists but that moment. In this space of freedom, they can make the transformational journey from unconsciousness to consciousness. Then they can feel that they are the source of true inner beauty.

CHAPTER TWO

THE BASICS OF TCM

Heaven has the sun and moon, humans have two eyes . . . Heaven has thunder and lightning, humans have sound and speech; Heaven has wind and rain, humans have joy and anger . . . Heaven has winter and summer, humans have hot and cold . . . Heaven has morning and evening, humans go to sleep and awake.

—Huang Di Nei Jing,
or The Yellow Emperor's Classic of Internal Medicine

I am descended from a great tradition of learning about the human body, mind and soul that is thousands of years old, and informed by the wisdom of the Taoist philosophers. They saw in each human being a microcosm of the universe. When we live according to the laws of nature, we live in harmony and health. When we resist the laws of nature, we can become imbalanced, and the result can be illness, disease or premature death.

In TCM, the starting point is always to evaluate the state of a person's health and well-being through many indicators. Is the person's energy flowing properly? What is going on in the person's life? Does the person eat, dress and sleep according to the seasons and in harmony with nature? What is happening in this person's body, mind, soul and life to provide an opportunity for disease? How can I support my patients' ability to heal themselves by achieving balance within their bodies and their beings?

Like the world itself, human beings have seasons in their lives. We would not wear heavy winter gear in the burning summer sun, or think to plant a garden in the snow. From birth to death, we must accept and honour the seasons in our lives and adapt to changing conditions in order to live consciously in the moment. Time and again, I see the suffering in those who refuse to accept the seasonal nature of their lives.

YIN AND YANG
阴阳 *(yīn yáng)*
In nature as in life, all things contain two opposite and complementary aspects or forces: hot and cold, male and female, dark and light, active and passive. This idea has been captured beautifully in the Chan poem "The Identity of Relative and Absolute," by Shih-tou:

> *Within light there is darkness,*
> *but do not try to understand that darkness.*
> *Within darkness there is light,*
> *but do not look for that light.*
> *Light and darkness are a pair,*
> *like the foot before and the foot behind in walking.*
> *Each thing has its own intrinsic value*
> *and is related to everything else in function and position.*
> *Ordinary life fits the absolute as a box and its lid.*
> *The absolute works together with the relative,*
> *like two arrows meeting in mid air.*

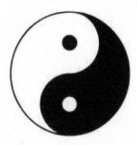

No modern graphic artist has been able to improve on the succinct and eloquent ancient Chinese symbol for Yin Yang.

Yin means "the shadowy side of the mountain" and is generally associated with shade, cold, contraction, the moon, water, inactivity, the feminine and matter. *Yang* means "the sunny side of the mountain" and is associated with brightness, heat, expansion, the sun, fire, activity, the masculine and energy. The ancient and universally recognized symbol for Yin Yang conveys a world of understanding: that day turns to night, that mothers give birth to children, that men and women each contain a little bit of the opposite gender's energy in their makeup to bring balance to their natures. Mothers are courageous and fathers are tender with their children. The moon shines bright in the night, and trees provide shade and coolness to protect us from the heat of the sun. Yin and Yang are essential to the understanding of TCM, and of life itself.

THE THREE TREASURES: JING, QI AND SHEN
精气神 *(jīng qì shén)*

The patients I see every day live in a turbulent world of constant pressures—at home, at work and in the broader society. These forces affect their ability to live in harmony with the three levels of energy known in TCM as the Three Treasures. They are Jing, or Essence; Qi, the natural life-bearing energy of the universe; and Shen, meaning spirit or mind. My first book, *Reflections of the Moon on Water,* was rooted primarily in Jing, the essence and historical origin of TCM. In that book, I tried to help readers understand how to preserve the fundamental assets that we receive from nature and our parents. In this book, we will emphasize Qi and its flow. If Qi moves smoothly and is properly balanced, this manifests in our largest organ, the skin, which glows with health and beauty from the inside out.

Jing 精

Jing, or Essence, is the substance that distinguishes living beings from inorganic things. It represents the life force we inherit from our parents that joins together at the time of conception—our genetic blueprint, if you will. It makes sense, then, that the Chinese character for Jing, 精, also means "sperm."

Jing represents the inexorable passage of time through us, in a movement that is so slow that we can only truly feel it in moments of reflection and contemplation. It governs how we develop, grow and decline over time. When we look back on our lives from the vantage point of old age, we can see its effect on our life cycle. Each person's prenatal or congenital Essence is unique, and predetermines how he or she will grow and develop. Postnatal Essence works with prenatal Essence to compose the overall Essence of a person. It comes from food and from the constantly changing physical, emotional and mental stimulation in a person's environment.

While we must make the best of our genetic inheritance, TCM places great emphasis on how we act to best preserve and enhance this genetic inheritance. This means taking care of ourselves through diet, exercise and generally avoiding the abuse of our bodies, minds and spirits.

Qi 气

Qi is the life force itself. The Chinese character for Qi, 气, comes from the idea of steam rising from cooking rice. This embodies the transformative character of Qi, as well as the material (rice) and immaterial (steam) states. It is often difficult to translate Chinese concepts perfectly into Western thought, but the closest equivalent to Qi is pure energy. As the great scholar Manfred Porkert said, "When Chinese thinkers are unwilling or unable to fix the quality of an energetic phenomenon, the character Qi 气 inevitably flows from their brushes."

If Qi were plotted on a continuum from heavy to light, it would form rocks and earth, then liquids, and finally, in its most ethereal form, the breath that animates animals and human beings. While this may be a foreign way for people raised in the Western tradition to look at themselves, Chinese practitioners have been harmonizing the flow of Qi through their patients for more than three millennia.

Qi moves through the body via a network of pathways called Meridians. It is essential to produce Blood, which in the broader TCM definition refers not only to the fluid that moves through our blood vessels but also to the energetic quality that activates Blood to nourish and circulate through our bodies.

Qi is so important to the functioning of the human body that all of its manifestations show up both internally and externally. Disruptions in the flow of Qi in the Lung and Large Intestine are most likely to manifest as skin disorders. For example, someone with asthma will also have psoriasis; someone with diverticulitis will also have severe eczema.

Qi moves up and down, and in and out, in a cycle that balances different functions: promoting energy to operate the body's activities; warming the body and keeping it at a constant temperature; consolidating the body's Organs and retaining or expelling bodily fluids such as sweat, urine, saliva and ejaculate as needed. It transforms ingested substances into Essence, vital energy, or waste products such as urine, stools or exhaled breath. The balance of all these activities and functions is necessary to good health; imbalances lead to illness and disease.

Shen 神

Shen, 神, is the most subtle of the Three Treasures. It is timeless and formless. When the earthly form, the body, dies, the spirit remains. Perhaps the Western idea that comes closest to it is consciousness, which engages the mind and the spirit. When Qi and Jing are vital, healthy and flowing well, our spiritual health can flourish. As human beings, we feel the need to connect with others and to care for the world around us. Our capacity to be creative and curious, to feel a deep sense of awareness and meaning, to make decisions based on moral values—these are all aspects of Shen.

When people practise a caring profession, such as medicine or teaching or policing—they are drawing on Shen. When a person decides to plant a tree whose shade will be enjoyed only by her grandchildren, she is demonstrating that her Shen is alive and vital. Shen is the human being's capacity to be "an initiator, a participant, and a guardian of the universe."*

In Chinese tradition, you are healthy when your Three Treasures—Jing, Qi and Shen—are all aligned.

THE ZANG-FU ORGANS, 脏腑 (zàng fǔ)

TCM's way of classifying the body's Organ networks, or systems, encompasses the terms used in Western medicine but extends beyond them. *Zang* refers to "Yin" Organs (the Liver, Heart, Spleen, Lung and Kidneys), which are paired with *Fu*, or "Yang," Organs (the Gallbladder, Small Intestine, Stomach, Large Intestine and Urinary Bladder, respectively). Each pair is linked to a sense organ, such as the eyes and ears, as well as specific tissues in the body. For example, the Liver ensures the smooth movement of Qi and Blood, stores the Blood, governs the tendons and nourishes the eyes. If this seems counterintuitive, think of the ways in which seemingly unrelated symptoms appear, such as the yellowing of the whites of the eyes that accompanies liver diseases such as jaundice and hepatitis.

Similarly, the Lung (Yin) is paired with the Large Intestine (Yang), and together they govern the skin. This is why you will frequently see that people who suffer from psoriasis also have breathing allergies or asthma.

---

* Tu Wei-ming, "Pain and Suffering in Confucian Self-Cultivation," *Philosophy East and West* (1984): 385.

CAUSES OF THE ABSENCE OF HARMONY

TCM explains the absence of harmony through three catego-
ries of causes: Interior Causes, Exterior Causes and Neither
Exterior nor Interior Causes. These factors are disruptive to the
balance of the Three Treasures within the body, lowering its
immunity and the capacity to fight disease.

TABLE 1: EXTERIOR, INTERIOR AND NEITHER EXTERIOR NOR INTERIOR
      CAUSES OF DISEASE

EXTERIOR CAUSES	**Six Excesses** • Cold • Wind • Heat or Fire • Dampness • Dryness • Summer Heat
INTERIOR CAUSES	**Seven Emotions** • Joy • Anger • Anxiety • Obsession, over-pensiveness • Sadness • Horror • Fear
NEITHER EXTERIOR NOR INTERIOR CAUSES	• Too much or too little physical exertion • Lack of sexual activity, frequent pregnancies • Diet • Moderation in and timing of consumption • Nutritious foods • Constitution • Trauma

Exterior Causes of Disharmony

The Exterior Causes of disharmony are also known as the Six Excesses: Cold, Wind, Heat or Fire, Dampness, Dryness and Summer Heat. The ancient wisdom that your mother shared in your childhood—"Dress warmly, keep your feet dry"—is rooted in the reality that these pathogenic factors are related to climate. We should always dress appropriately for the weather, regardless of whether it is typical for the time of year. This is increasingly a factor with climate change. In Canada, we have begun to see mild Januarys and strange, chilly Junes.

Dryness and Dampness are also important conditions to note—we should make sure to keep up our intake of liquids and stay dry when it rains. Some of my patients find that the icy blast of air conditioners gives them stiff necks in the summer. I treat them with acupuncture and tui na treatments to reopen the flow of Qi in the Meridians that have been blocked by Dampness or Cold—and I advise them to wear a scarf in any air-conditioned environment. The higher the quality and the quantity of Qi in our bodies, the more resistance we have to these Exterior Causes of disharmony.

The number of my patients who present symptoms of psoriasis or eczema always rises dramatically over the long Toronto winter, when their skin is so rarely exposed to the sun. My patient Frances, like many others, suffered from unbearable itching, scaly skin and shedding all winter long, due to the dry artificial heat indoors. This condition caused an imbalance in her internal Yin Yang, and she suffered from excessive heat in her body.

I made sure Frances drank a lot of water, and I rebalanced her body using TCM techniques and supplements. Over a period of several years, the condition became less severe and lasted a shorter period of time, until she no longer experienced it.

Interior Causes of Disharmony

The Interior Causes of disharmony are our seven emotions: joy, anger, anxiety, obsession, sadness, horror and fear. We may be adversely affected by any excessive experience of these emotions over a period of time. We may experience these emotions deeply, but keeping them in balance over time is important to avoid compromising our health. We now know from extensive research that stressful life events, such as the death of a spouse or living in a war-torn region, can push people into illness and disease. As a result, a whole branch of Western medicine known as psychoneuroimmunology now exists to help healing processes through relaxation, meditation and visualization.

TCM considers that problems of emotional and mental health are also physical, arising from an energy imbalance in an Organ system. Emotions flow according to Qi; we experience significant problems when there is a blockage. The *Nei Jing,* considered the founding text of TCM, says: "It is known that all diseases arise from the upset of Qi: Anger pushes the Qi up, joy makes the Qi slacken, grief disperses the Qi, fear brings the Qi down, terror confuses the Qi, and anxiety causes the Qi to stagnate. Anger harms the Liver, joy the Heart, anxiety the Spleen, grief the Lung and fear the Kidneys."

In TCM, tears are not solely a manifestation of sorrow or distress. They can also come with an overflow of joy. In this case, they show the body's attempts to balance an excess of happiness, which can add stress to the Heart over time. Excessive sadness and grief can lead to disharmony in the flow of Lung Qi and result in a cold, asthma or psoriasis, since skin is the tissue governed by the Lung. If you worry too much, this may block Spleen Qi and result in digestive problems or excessive menstrual bleeding.

Women are particularly prone to experiencing gynecological disorders that result from blocked Qi and interconnected emotional, physical and mental ailments. This integration of emotional and spiritual with physical well-being is deeply rooted in TCM as it was practised historically. Modern China has moved away from this notion with the advent of an ideology based on materialism. I sense that this may be changing as China moves toward globalization and a renewed interest in TCM as it existed centuries ago, but when I was a student and a young practitioner in China, it was not common to discuss emotional problems with patients.

When I moved to Canada, I realized that my patients had a deep need to talk about their lives, and that their psychological health was crucial in healing their bodies. I therefore underwent psychotherapy myself, in order to understand how my patients think and react to events in their lives. This was extremely beneficial, as it caused me to discover my own suffering and struggles to be loved and accepted. It gave me common ground with my patients and has been enormously helpful to me in finding the right treatments to advance their holistic well-being.

Alice, who I told you about in Chapter One, provides a classic example of how excessive emotion can disturb the body's balance and tip it into illness. She and her husband had accepted their son's diabetes and helped him live a normal life into young adulthood. Alice's health was in balance and she was happy.

This changed when their son was in his late twenties. While working in a tropical country, he became very ill. He made it back to Canada, but by the time he got here, he was running a dangerously high fever. For weeks, no one could diagnose his illness. During this time, Alice began to suffer from psoriasis— at first just a few spots on her hands and legs. But then it spread very rapidly, until nearly all of her body (but not her face) was covered with painful red patches.

For a description of psoriasis, and recipes for herbal remedies, both topical and internal, see page 156.

By the time Alice came to me, she was in extreme discomfort. She could no longer wear her normal clothes, at work, at home or in bed. She had seen two different dermatologists, and their various prescriptions and creams required her to cover herself up at all times with clothing that quickly became soaked and stained with grease spots. Her always supportive husband was away on business much of the time, and she was almost relieved to be sleeping alone, given the circumstances. None of the creams helped; the psoriasis kept getting worse, even when Alice's son returned to health.

Like many patients, Alice came to our clinic as a last resort, because all of the obvious channels had failed. She was puzzled about the virulence of her problem because she had handled her previous illnesses successfully. The influx of high emotion caused by her son's crisis had broken through the protective barrier she had erected at the time of his diabetes diagnosis two decades before, and all of the earlier fears had snowballed with the new ones: she was terrified of losing her son, even while she recognized that her feelings were irrational. Her emotions were out of control—she could not sleep or keep her food down—and the skin problems had followed hard on the heels of the emotional crisis.

Her pulse and tongue told me that Alice was suffering from indigestion. "I'm nauseous and I've lost twenty pounds in just three weeks," she told me. Acupuncture, herbs, tui na therapy and a diet with more protein helped to stabilize Alice quickly. To calm her emotions, she began to meditate. Three months later, the psoriasis crisis had completely subsided.

Neither Exterior nor Interior Causes of Disharmony

The causes of disharmony that are Neither Exterior nor Interior include diet, physical exertion, sexual activity and trauma, which are discussed more fully in the following chapters.

Diet. In TCM, the body's balance depends on consuming the right amounts of various types of foods. For example, too much salt can cause a Kidney imbalance, leading to high blood pressure, water retention and headaches. Too many sweets can cause Dampness in the Spleen, leading to poor digestion, irregular bowel movements and swelling. TCM also uses food as medicine, particularly medicinal herbs, which help to balance the organ systems, and food herbs, which help to strengthen and support the body, as well as prevent disease.

TCM's use of customized blends of herbs suited to each patient's particular makeup and situation contrasts with the Western medical practice of designing drugs for conditions and then giving them to everyone who displays that condition. The diet recommended by a TCM practitioner will vary according to the weather and the patient's internal and external condition. Above all, TCM preaches moderation and balance in diet, based on each person's basic constitution, current health and climatic factors.

Foods are also classified by flavours and affinities for specific Organs. For example, sour foods (vinegar, lemons) are associated with the Liver; salty foods (celery, seaweed) with the Kidneys; bitter foods (dark green leafy vegetables, bitter melon) with the Heart; and pungent foods (tofu, garlic) with the Lung. Foods are also categorized by temperature as it relates to their energetic qualities: Hot and Warm foods include pumpkin, ginger, onions and chicken, for example, while Neutral, Cool or Cold foods include barley, lettuce, tomato and duck among others. I will discuss diet more fully in Chapter Six, which is on nutrition and lifestyle.

Physical Exertion. For optimal health, we need healthy sleep and rest, not overworking or overtaxing the body physically, emotionally and mentally. Exercise is very important to keep the Qi and Blood moving. But overly forceful and vigorous exercise can actually damage the body through injuries and disharmony caused by excessive demand on the Qi and the Blood to sustain the specific muscles and tendons used.

I see dozens of cases a week where patients are simply working too much, too long and under too much pressure. The obsessive nature of North American business and the unreasonable demands on people in the workplace lead to many illnesses. Some people also carry this obsessiveness over into the home, making themselves sick with obligations and driving their children crazy by overscheduling them into every kind of lesson and activity imaginable, with no time for spontaneous play. Others show up with chronic injuries from running or high-impact aerobics, damaging their bodies in the drive for perfection.

Balance in physical activity is necessary throughout life, but it is particularly important during periods when our bodies are under stress or working hard: when our Heavenly Water is flowing (menstruation), when we are "Ripening the Fruit" (pregnant), when we are breastfeeding, when we are ill, when we are experiencing emotional difficulties, or when we are undergoing the physical and spiritual changes of Second Spring (menopause).

Clouds and Rain.

Clouds and Rain. In TCM, sexual energy is a powerful force for healing and for physical and mental health. There are many ways to cultivate this energy. While this cultivation does not depend on sexual activity, orgasms do promote the smooth flow of Qi throughout the organ systems. Sexual energy is as important as food in the balance of Yin and Yang that promotes health and longevity.

The ancient Taoists called the exchange of bodily fluids and energy that happens during the sex act 云雨 yún-yu, or "clouds and rain." Sexual activity is a source of pleasure and fulfillment that promotes longevity. When men and women cultivate their sexual energy, there is no reason why they cannot continue to be sexually active throughout their entire lives. I will explore sexual energy more fully in Chapter Four, where I discuss relationships.

A SUMMARY OF THE BASIC CONCEPTS OF THE TCM APPROACH TO HEALTH

Holistic and Causal

TCM looks at the whole person: the whole body, mind and spirit, as well as the surrounding circumstances and factors that may be playing a role in his or her state of health. It takes for granted the possibility that symptoms are arising from a remotely located cause. It views disease as an imbalance in the body's natural harmony and seeks to identify and treat its root cause rather than just the symptoms.

Preventive and Natural

TCM watches over the body's natural ability to heal and balance itself, and seeks to treat imbalances before they trigger physical symptoms. It works in partnership with the patient, who must take responsibility for his or her own health by adopting an appropriate lifestyle: diet, exercise and meditation or other techniques to support mental health and inner peace. It tries to avoid triggering new problems with preventive measures, such as taking an Aspirin every day for heart health at the risk of irritating the digestive system.

Individual

Every patient who enters a TCM process receives a customized diagnosis and treatment. Because TCM views symptoms as only one element in an integrated diagnosis that will vary widely according to a patient's personal state of being, energy flows and balances, each treatment protocol will be highly specific to that patient. This approach differs sharply from that of Western medicine. The ancient Taoist texts tell us that the sages of the time lived long, healthy lives by living in harmony with the vital energy that is present in the human body and in the universe, thereby preventing disease over long periods of time.

HARMONY IN BODY AND MIND: THE SOURCE OF INNER BEAUTY

When asked to describe a beautiful person, almost anyone will give you an answer that includes signs of balanced health according to TCM: bright, clear eyes; glowing skin; healthy, shiny hair; smooth, unridged nails; and moist lips.

Throughout the ages, and certainly by the time of Cicero, the eyes have been described as the window to the soul. A person with bright, clear eyes may indeed be displaying a beautiful soul, but in TCM, he or she is also showing a clean Liver. When the Liver is engorged or obstructed—this can happen easily when large quantities of alcohol, red meat and coffee are consumed, for example—the eyes will be cloudy.

Aside from moderation in all things, it helps to cleanse the Liver with sour foods and liquids, which is why I drink

Inner beauty radiates . . . There are two sides to beauty: the physical—we can't be oblivious to that because of all the instant media all around us—and the spiritual and emotional beauty that you combine for the gestalt that makes you who you are. The inside influences the outside, and the outside influences the inside. If you're at peace with yourself, you're happy, and you find meaning in your life.

—ALBERTA CEFIS, PATIENT, ARTS VOLUNTEER AND MULTINATIONAL EXECUTIVE a glass of lemon water every morning. The Liver is the body's largest Organ for detoxification, and it is very important to keep it working well and freely.

In TCM beautiful, healthy skin is often compared to jade. Although this may sound strange to Western ears, it makes sense to Chinese people because of the stone's place in history. For centuries, people who lived in China's wealthy households and imperial courts used jade in many ways: they ate it, they wore it, they sucked on it and they had it placed in their burial chambers. Jade has long been used in TCM to calm the soul, maintain healthy blood circulation and "moisten" the Heart and Lung to protect and lubricate body tissues. The ancient Chinese used it to prevent and cure disease and to slow the aging process.

Jade is seen, metaphorically, as a box for the storage of Qi, keeping Yin and Yang in balance. Today we know that the stone contains a number of mineral elements (zinc, iron, copper, manganese, cobalt, selenium, chromium, titanium, lithium, calcium and sodium), and it is possible that wearing the stone on the skin supplements the body's dietary requirements for these minerals. TCM also holds that jade can facilitate a discharge of excess elements from the body.

No wonder, then, that beautiful, healthy skin is so often compared to jade: translucent and protective, acting as the body's living, breathing membrane between the inner Organs and the outside world, the skin is beautifully designed to guard against external Toxins. But even small forms of trauma—anything that itches and provokes persistent scratching, for example, such as eczema and fungal conditions or flea and lice bites—can damage or remove the first layer of skin and allow Toxins to invade. External Causes can weaken the Qi and create internal Heat Toxins that obstruct the channels and network vessels.

The skin also displays internal imbalances of the Five Organs, especially of the Lung and the Large Intestine. Diabetic patients are particularly vulnerable to skin conditions because blood flow to their skin is poor.

The movement of Qi manifests clearly in the skin, especially when there is a blockage in one of the Meridians. Itchy, red or broken skin broadcasts a clear message to the TCM practitioner. I can often tell just by looking at a patient that he or she is experiencing Stomach, Kidney, Liver or Spleen problems.

You should not be afraid when your skin has a problem: your skin is speaking to you, encouraging you to take care of your needs by seeking treatment to release the Toxins that are causing the imbalance in your body. Skin problems are the language through which your body tells you that you have a blockage of Qi that needs to be fixed.

We do not always think of the hair as a part of the skin, but it is. Beautiful, healthy Chinese hair is like ebony silk, and this is how we think of it poetically. Such hair clearly demonstrates inner health and beauty, its richness and shine showing strong Kidney Qi, a wealth of Blood and adequate, balanced moisture in the body.

Weak, dull hair, or hair that is falling out, immediately alerts a TCM practitioner of a Kidney imbalance that needs to be addressed. All patients are sensitive to these signs, whether they are men or women, young or old—everyone sees hair as part of their external beauty, and many are self-conscious about the state of

Inner beauty is cultivated by the individual. It's about awareness of one's thoughts, their consciousness, their essence, and bringing that into the world through one's body . . . What is more beautiful than a woman who walks down a street knowing exactly who she is? Who is more beautiful than the woman who knows herself and carries an open heart? A mother. A lover. A dancer. Grace. These women who carry all of this with them in every moment, inside, outside.

—DAVID BATTISTELLA, SCREEN-WRITER, FILM PRODUCER AND PATIENT their hair. Patients who are experiencing hair problems are often anxious to consult and obtain help to address them.

When a person is healthy, calm and self-confident, her Qi radiates and she is beautiful.

In TCM, maintaining harmony is the primary way of achieving well-being. Our physical, emotional and spiritual selves— the three levels of energy described as the Three Treasures, Jing, Qi and Shen—must be in balance. A strong, healthy body helps us to stabilize our emotional lives and deepen our spiritual selves. These aspects of health are intimately interconnected, and we must be proactive in maintaining them. Diet, lifestyle, wisdom in our actions toward ourselves and others are all essential elements in preventing disease and promoting health. No medical professional can overcome the effects of consistent bad decisions on our part.

> Medicine can only cure curable disease, and then not always.
> —*Chinese proverb*

TCM TREATMENT

> The best doctors are Dr. Diet, Dr. Quiet and Dr. Merryman.
> —*Chinese proverb*

TCM uses three broad treatment techniques, all of which can apply to skin conditions: acupuncture, tui na and herbs for both internal and external use. All three of these approaches play a role in rebalancing the body.

Acupuncture, an essential technique of TCM, uses fine needles to stimulate or calm the flow of Qi through the body, to restore and balance its energy and return it to health. We think of health as a state of balance in which Blood, which is Yin, and Qi, which is Yang, harmonize into a unitary whole.

The body has fourteen Meridians, or channels. In a healthy body, Qi travels through all of them. When there is a blockage in a Meridian, symptoms develop. Inserting a fine acupuncture needle into specific body points along the Meridians is an effective way to ensure that the Qi can once again travel smoothly. In some instances, the relief is immediate. In others, treatments can take more time.

Tui na, or massage therapy, is also designed to promote movement of Qi along the Meridian pathways, treat musculoskeletal and soft tissue problems and balance the body. Originally developed for treating children, it is now commonly used to promote healing among adults. The practitioner uses his or her hands, thumbs, elbows and whatever level of pressure is required along the Meridians and on acupressure points.

TCM prescribes herbs as food and as medicine, both for internal and external use. These are integral to balancing the functioning of the Organ systems. Food herbs are part of the daily diet, building strength, preventing disease and supporting overall good health. Medicinal herbs include a wide range of plant extracts and mineral and animal products, all sourced from nature. A herb prescribed for a specific Organ will both resonate with it energetically and influence it biochemically. The resultant smooth movement of Qi within that Organ system benefits other Organs as well.

I have compiled a glossary of the herbs I use in my practice, which

When a patient first comes to see me, I take on 50 per cent of the responsibility for his health, while he has 50 per cent. But eventually, he takes 95 per cent and I take 5. I don't live with him, shop with him, and make sure he eats, sleeps and exercises. He comes here once every two weeks, but the rest of the time the responsibility is his.

—XIAOLAN

begins on page 212. If you are interested in procuring these herbs, the glossary will ensure that there is no mistake in what you buy: it offers the English name, Latin botanical name, Chinese characters and romanized Pinyin pronunciation of the Chinese name for each herb. This way, if you purchase the herbs from a Chinese herbalist who does not speak English, you can ensure that you are getting the right product. This is important, as some of these herbs can have a powerful effect on the body. Combining the herbs also results in different properties, and it is important to observe the proportions and preparation procedures in the reference section, which begins on page 77.

Like all TCM practitioners, I combine herbs to produce remedies that are specially designed for a patient's unique constitution and emotional and physical health, as well as his or her environment. TCM herbs are also available in packaged doses based on classical formulas that are strictly regulated. While the use of these products is less flexible than the traditional customized herbal formulas, it provides tremendous advantages in convenience and consistency of ingredients, and I use a great deal of them in my practice.

At the heart of TCM is prevention of disease. For example, during pregnancy, a woman's husband or her mother, or she herself, will prepare a herbal oil and use it to massage her belly. This beautiful purple oil, Purple Rejuvenation Massage Oil or 紫草根油 (zǐ cǎo gēn yóu), will keep the skin healthy and resilient and prevent stretch marks (see recipe on page 188). The homemade preparation has a multitude of uses: preventing diaper rash in babies, treating cradle cap, preventing and treating cracked nipples during breastfeeding, and all manner of skin dryness and itchy conditions. There are many other herbal preparations and oils that we use to prevent and treat skin conditions. I have selected the ones I believe will be most useful to you for inclusion in this book.

CHAPTER THREE

THE BREATH OF LIFE

呼吸 *(Hū Xī)*

Breathing properly is an amazing, totally inexpensive way to come home to the now, where nature really wants us to live.

—*Paul Winter*

"Ten to ten!" From the time I was seven years old, for me and for all Chinese children, this was the daily call after the second period of class. It was the signal that every single person in the school had to be outside right away for twenty minutes of exercise. This period was not the free-form recess of the West! It was the time to follow a precise set of movements to stretch our muscles and to practise healthy breathing.

"The nose is for breathing, the mouth is for eating." We were constantly reminded that healthy breathing comes through the nose, where the small hairs called cilia act like scrubbers to clean and filter the air before sending it down a long, warm, alkaline passage, preparing it ideally for the Lung to breathe in and out.

"呼吸, 呼吸 (hū xī, hū xī)," we would say as we practised our breathing. The first syllable (pronounced *hoo*) emphasizes the importance of exhaling. It is the beginning of life and its end: the newborn's first cry of protest as it squeezes out of its mother's womb, and the very last act of every dying person. But the quality of breathing between birth and death will affect every person's longevity and quality of life.

Knowing so well from early childhood that breathing is life itself, imagine my surprise to find that among my first Canadian patients, four out of five had no concept of proper breathing. They habitually breathed through their mouths, sending cold, unfiltered, acidic air into their poor, abused Lung. Furthermore, most of them had absolutely no idea that they were doing this. When I raised it with them, they were startled: isn't breathing something totally automatic? They had never stopped to think about it. This concerned me, because these bad breathing habits were causing multiple health problems for my patients: vulnerability to allergies, colds, asthma, bloated Stomach, mental fatigue, insomnia, sleep apnea and many other illnesses.

Without the lifelong training in hu-xi, my Western patients had been influenced by moments of fear in childhood: holding their breath and inhaling at the first opportunity. They had come to think of inhaling as the most important part of breathing. They became easily afraid of not having enough air. They had never developed the habit of exhaling fully. Many of them found that their breathing grew increasingly shallow over time, with a corresponding reduction in Lung capacity and in vital energy—and they had no idea why.

I also noticed that some of my patients were so focused on listening to what I said to them—perhaps because of my accent!—that they actually held their breath while I was talking. I still find myself constantly reminding them to breathe!

Once I had discovered this problem, I instituted a practice that continues to this day in my clinic. Each time a patient lies down on one of our tables, my colleagues and I begin the hour-long treatment by using essential oils of eucalyptus and peppermint to open up ears and nostrils. We evaluate the patient's breathing. Is it weak or strong? Deep or shallow? Ragged or smooth? The answers to these questions tell us a great deal about the state of the patient's health.

Charlotte came to me, as many patients do, in crisis. Just three months before, she had been healthy and normal. Now, coming to my clinic for the first time, she had developed both asthma and eczema, and she was gasping for air. The more she gasped, the more afraid she was that the next breath would not come. She was using a steroid inhaler to breathe and cortisone cream for her skin. And she was getting steadily worse.

The trigger for all this had been a two-part tragedy: her beloved father had suffered a crippling stroke and her best friend had died unexpectedly. She caught a persistent cold, which settled into her Lung and then developed into asthma. The overwhelming stress of her father's sudden dependence on her and the grief over her friend's death had snowballed to damage Charlotte's health severely.

First, as she lay on her back, I used the eucalyptus and peppermint oils to open up her nose. I explained to her that if her Lung did not let go of the dirty air that would carry carbon dioxide and Toxins out of her body, she could not make room for the fresh air that would provide her with healing and revitalizing oxygen. "Imagine," I told her, "that this room was full of boxes and I asked you to lie down. You would protest—you would tell me that there is no room here to lie down. Your Lung is no different. If you don't make room for fresh air, you can't inhale. Exhaling is always the first step to proper breathing."

Gently, I asked Charlotte to breathe with me. Slowly, we began practising longer and deeper exhales. I put a needle into the acupuncture point we call 鸠尾 (jiū wěi), which means "dovetail"—the movement of breathing resembles a bird's body in flight, and the acupuncture point is located right at the diaphragm. I stimulated the needle constantly to produce a sensation that would help her to focus on her diaphragm, and asked her at the same time to exhale while squeezing the point around the needle. Gradually, each exhale became easier and her bronchial wheezing subsided. She stopped panicking and began to relax. By the end of the first one-hour treatment, her breathing was much improved. I sent her home with herbs and the following exercise:

This exercise is made up of three consecutive breaths. Lie down with your feet flat on the floor, your knees bent and your head comfortably resting. Use a small pillow if that feels right. Your body should be completely relaxed so that you can focus exclusively on your breathing.

Next, put your hands on the jiu wei point and exhale completely. Then, inhale halfway, and exhale fully again. Repeat. On the third breath, open up your chest and inhale deeply and fully, then exhale completely again. Do ten repetitions of this exercise, three times a day.

Charlotte took my recommendations seriously. She took her herbs daily and she did the exercises conscientiously. Her asthma was recent, and acute rather than chronic. Her Lung had not had time to sustain much damage. Her recovery was therefore much quicker and easier than it would have been had her asthma been chronic. Within a week, she no longer felt the need for the inhaler. Within a month, she was fully recovered: her skin was back to normal, her allergies and asthma had completely disappeared. Her anxieties over her father had dissipated, and she was able to be cheerful again. To this day, Charlotte says she was cured by "magic breathing."

THE ROLE OF AIR IN BUILDING QI 气

We are born with vital energy from our parents, which is stored by the Kidney for use as needed. The Spleen transforms the food and water we consume, while the Lung takes nutrition from the air that we breathe. These three sources combine to create the Qi that animates us and gives us life.

While the Lung administers breathing, the Kidneys play a

role in the body's absorption and use of the air. This is why an imbalance in the Kidneys may trigger respiratory problems such as asthma, or cause a blockage that prevents a person from over-coming fear or grief.

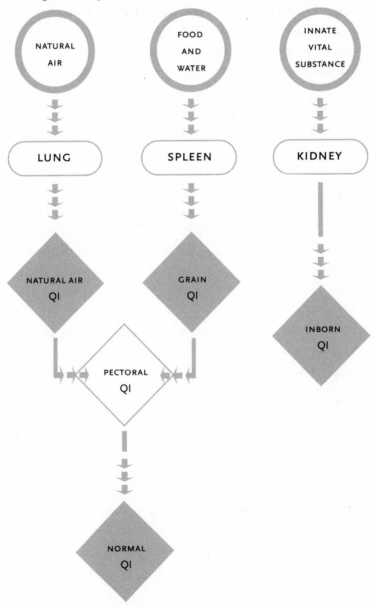

A person with healthy Lung Qi speaks well and freely, with moderate and rhythmic breathing, while someone with a Deficiency will have garbled speech, a weak voice and shortness of breath, as well as a quick, irregular, weak or scattered pulse. Often, a Lung Deficiency will lead to Heart problems. This is why a patient suffering from chronic bronchitis will tend to develop pulmonary heart disease: shortness of breath, a low voice, palpitations, a purplish face and a running or intermittent pulse.

THE ESSENCE OF MOVEMENT: THE DIAPHRAGM
隔膜 *(gé mó)*

Richard looks like the healthiest young man you could imagine. He is muscular—perhaps even "muscle-bound," as a result of constant training and a mountain-climbing habit he can afford to indulge. His appearance, however, is deceptive. When he first walked into my clinic, he told me he had experienced three bouts of pneumonia in a row over the previous six months. He was still on a course of antibiotics because he was so afraid that it would come back.

He lay down on the treatment table, and I put my finger on his jiu wei point. I asked him to breathe down to my finger. He inhaled through his mouth, because his nose was stuffed up. No matter how hard he tried, at that moment he could not bring the breath down to my finger. The hard muscles he had built were so rigid that they were trapping him into shallow breathing.

Most of us take breathing for granted because it is an involuntary act that happens by itself throughout our lives. The truth is, however, that the vast majority of people are only using about 30 per cent of their Lung capacity—and therefore, they are producing far less Qi than they should. All the tissues of the body need oxygen to heal from injuries and to thrive, especially the brain. Someone who is not breathing to capacity is also not achieving his or her potential. Imagine the increase in energy, vitality, alertness, competence and good general health that would result if only they knew how to increase the use of the easily available capacity that they already have!

Many people wrongly believe that getting enough air into the lungs is the most important element of breathing. But if the lungs are not fully expelling the waste-carrying air when they exhale, fresh air with nutritional and healing oxygen cannot enter the Lung. We see in weak patients with Lung disease that a chronic inability to exhale completely results in stagnant air accumulating in the Lung, and increasingly shallow breathing. In severe Lung diseases such as cancer and emphysema, this can eventually result in serious infections and death.

The first step in improving Lung capacity is to understand the role of the diaphragm, the control centre for all of the body's energy and movement. It is a wonderful example of the beautiful design of the human body, and its innate intelligence.

Few people realize how large and powerful the diaphragm is. This strong, dome-shaped muscle actually occupies a whole "floor" in our bodies. This is why healthy breathing happens in the whole thorax, in three dimensions, not just in one vertical channel. Like an elevator, the diaphragm muscle rises and falls with normal breathing, which begins with the exhale. Only when the diaphragm has pushed out the stale air from our lungs does fresh air rush back in to take its place. This involuntary movement makes breathing the exact opposite of what most people perceive it to be: we do not need to gasp to suck air in, but rather to exhale properly to let air out. The diaphragm automatically takes care of bringing in the fresh air. Breathing problems are almost always caused by a weak ability to exhale.

In addition to its all-important role in breathing, the diaphragm maintains a perfect seal between the upper and lower torso, thereby preventing infection from spreading between the abdominal and thoracic cavities. In moving up and down, it also massages all the torsal Organs in turn, preventing adhesions and keeping them free-moving and healthy.

When Richard realized that his serial pneumonia was linked to bad breathing, he worked with me to change it. He learned to breathe in three dimensions, using his diaphragm, his back muscles and abdomen to expand the amount of oxygen he was taking in. Eventually, he was able to breathe deeply enough to power all those big muscles he had built. After he began TCM treatments with us, he never had pneumonia again.

CONSCIOUS BREATHING AND JINGSHEN
精神 *(jīng shén)*

Breathing regularly and deeply, as well as exhaling completely to release waste from the body, has a direct effect on the health and well-being of a person's mind and spirit, known as *Jingshen* (精神).

Catharine, a young woman who wanted to be in a helping or healing profession, went through a difficult period at the age of twenty-three. Her university degree in psychology had been a disappointment and had not led to the path she was seeking. She was upset about her parents' recent divorce. After graduation, she moved to a remote rural area and continued to live a typical North American student lifestyle, surviving on beer and pizza.

In this small town, it was easy to meet people socially—everyone knew everyone. Catharine was fortunate to meet a woman whom she would think of as a catalyst for the rest of her life. The woman, a mother of three, lived a life of authenticity that Catharine admired. She sought advice from the woman, who told her that working on her breathing would help unblock her potential. They began regular sessions of what the woman called "Mahatma Breath Work." Over a period of a few months,

Catharine worked through her emotions and learned to detach them from the stories that had caused them. This allowed her not to remain stuck in these emotions, but to let them flow through her.

The breathing techniques gave her a safe place to become truly and authentically herself, and to centre herself in the moment. As a by-product of the process, she lost twenty-five pounds and began to feel lighter. She also realized that shallow breathing had been the trigger of her intense anxiety. Although these events happened many years ago, Catharine continues to use these breathing skills today to recentre herself and to remain healthy. Now that she has two children, she also uses breathing to work through her children's problems and anxieties, teaching them to breathe along with her.

As we have seen, bad breathing habits are deceptively and dangerously widespread—but of course this means that there is a huge opportunity to improve quality of life for many people simply by learning conscious breathing. Becoming aware of your breathing is a wonderful and simple way to begin to live alertly in the present moment. It stills a hyperactive brain and clears space for calm and consciousness. It can break patterns of anxiety and pain and open up opportunities to experience our own inner richness and the beauty that surrounds us.

As long as we are available and not overriding our natural instincts, our bodies actually manage breathing all by themselves. We do not need to provide hands-on direction, misinformed by destructive life experiences. We can just step back and watch—and it is wonderful what happens when we do.

It is never too late to begin incorporating conscious breathing into our daily routine—and it will change your life when you do. Everyone can afford to take ten minutes a day to lie down and think about nothing else but breathing.

The breath is mysterious and subtle, without shape or form. Once you pay attention to it, you will find that you become acutely alert but surprisingly peaceful. Your mind cannot race while you are concentrating on breathing in and breathing out. It is the beginning of an inner transformation.

A SIMPLE BREATHING EXERCISE AND A TOOL FOR LONGEVITY

The ancient secret of longevity is based on food and breathing—both key inputs to the making of Qi inside our bodies. In China, physical disciplines that encompass conscious breathing, such as Tai Chi, 太极 (tài jí), or Qi Gong, 气功 (qì gōng), are part of a daily routine considered essential to health and longevity.

The first step in being truly present in your life is to be conscious of your breathing. This fundamental act of life may seem very obvious, but believe me, most people never think about it. It is never too late to begin incorporating conscious breathing into your daily routine—and it will change your life when you do. The most wonderful thing about breathing exercises is that you can do them almost anywhere or any time—and you can do them sitting, standing or lying down. You don't need any special equipment or a club membership to begin a lifetime of conscious breathing. Just start now—you'll be so glad you did. Here is an exercise you should do every day of your life.

Breathe in deeply and slowly. Feel the air moving in and out of your body. Notice how your chest expands and your belly rises. Experience the feeling of your back muscles expanding and contracting. Exhale fully, contracting your belly. Observe your breathing, its depth, its rhythm and pattern. Is it even or ragged? Deep or shallow? Are you expelling all the air? Most people's breathing is artificially shallow, but when you begin to pay attention to it, you will find it deepening. You will also

become aware of the still point just after you finish exhaling, and before
you inhale once again.

Smooth, healthy breathing will cause the base of your rib cage to
expand gently in and out, like bird wings. Do your breathing
exercises when you can devote all your attention to them.
Becoming more aware of your breathing will help you reduce
the stress and tension that impedes the smooth flow of Qi in your
body—and this alone will improve your health and longevity.

If we can master breathing, we can create the space in our
lives to be in the moment, connected to our most authentic
selves. This is the key to health and inner beauty.

CHAPTER FOUR

RELATIONSHIPS: THE WEB OF LIFE

To understand your parents' love, bear your own children.
—*Chinese proverb*

When I first lived with my parents again after my life of freedom with my grandmother, we all found it very hard to adjust. I can only imagine how my mother must have felt, having been forced to leave her eight-month-old baby and returning to find a six-year-old stranger. At first, I wanted nothing to do with her and blamed her for removing me from my grandmother's house.

My mother's way of reconnecting with me involved a kind of wooing. She would tell me stories and sing to me, until I engaged with her, laughing and singing. To this day, singing feels to me like a wonderful expression of joy, which may explain my love of opera!

When I co-operated with her and learned new things—such as reading a story back to her—I was allowed to have a new book. The ritual of taking her hand and going with her to buy a new book every Saturday helped to take the edge off my grief at being separated from my beloved grandmother.

In my grandmother's house, time had no meaning. The hours passed in a fog of bliss, without my being aware of them. This was not acceptable to my father, who, in fairness, was also very concerned with my welfare in dangerous times. Once I was living with my parents again, my father would post a strict schedule, in writing, at the head of my bed. He expected me to rise at 7:00, brush my teeth and have breakfast at a specific time, and at all times he expected me to comply with his orders. At first, I was angered by this and refused to obey. He would put the schedule up and I would take it down. Day after day, he and I waged a war of attrition. We are both very strong-willed! For the first time in my life, I felt that I was being judged rather than accepted as I was.

One day at the table, when I was being particularly difficult and refusing to allow my brother to have some of my favourite food, my father punished me by hitting my hand and ordering me to stop this behaviour. The whole family was dumbstruck, as no one had ever laid a hand on me before. I was so shocked that I pushed myself away from the table and ran to my bed. This period was painful for me, and I have never forgotten how it felt to make the transition from "wild grass" to domesticated child.

I continue to think that self-confidence and authenticity are rooted in unconditional love in childhood. When I see my patients, both parents and children, I hope for them that they can teach their children without this painful process of domestication that changes how children relate to the world. Nurturing a sense of wonder and delight in children is an endless source of happiness for the whole family.

> Govern a family as you would cook a small fish—very gently.
> —*Chinese proverb*

Although my siblings were much older than me, we were still a relatively large family. By the time I was twenty-seven years old, China's one-child policy was an omnipresent reality in our lives. When I became pregnant with my son, the baby was considered extremely precious, not just because my whole family knew he would be my only child, but because twenty-seven was considered an advanced age for childbirth. Throughout my pregnancy—a condition that we call "Ripening the Fruit"—my husband and family took great care to help me conserve energy and remain healthy for the baby's birth. They would ensure that I got choice morsels of food; my husband would massage the skin on my belly carefully to help prevent stretch marks; and they all made sure that I got lots of rest.

On my arrival in North America, I was very surprised to see women of forty having a first child! Of course, whatever their age, the women who come to see me also think of their babies as very precious. But not all of them can enjoy the same kind of solicitous care that I had, making me feel always beautiful during this special time. I remember that I felt transformed by the growing feeling of unconditional love toward my unborn child, and nourished physically and in every other way throughout my pregnancy.

In China, a woman who gives birth is expected to rest completely for the following "Golden Month." The family rallies to ensure that she does absolutely nothing during that period except eat, feed her baby and sleep. This cocoon of love and protection truly gives her a great start as a new parent, and allows her to concentrate on regaining her strength and bonding with her newborn child. I was so privileged to experience this loving beginning to my son's life, and the nurturing that helped me recover from my Caesarean delivery and return to glowing health.

Unfortunately, there is no such tradition in North America, where I have even seen some of these forty-year-old mothers drag themselves back to the office within a few days of giving birth, leaving the newborn with a nanny! These mothers often end up in my clinic with classic symptoms of Qi and Blood deficiencies: exhaustion, hair loss, rough and irritated skin, and postpartum depression.

Recently, I had a conversation with two young women I know well—one whose pregnancy was gloriously happy, with a husband who never stopped telling her how beautiful she was throughout, and the other with a more difficult situation. While she was also very happy about her healthy and beautiful new baby, the pregnancy had been more stressful, as her husband found it impossible to maintain his normal attitude toward her sexual attractiveness during the pregnancy.

This meant she had to draw much more deeply on her personal resources to remain strong and confident of her inner beauty. This calm confidence is very important to maintaining a normal, healthy flow of Qi and supporting the baby's growth.

Families and friends can be of great help during pregnancy and childbirth, supporting the woman emotionally, but also in many practical ways that help her concentrate her energies on delivering and caring for a healthy, happy baby. Many women, as I did, take great comfort in having their own mothers in the house, making their favourite foods, keeping the household stable and focusing on the well-being of mother and child. This is when we begin to gain a deeper understanding of our parents' love and contribution to our lives.

Babies are my inspiration and my joy. In them, I see innocence and the precious possibilities of each life unfolding. In my images, I hope to convey a measure of the beauty that exists in all children.

—ANNE GEDDES, BABY PHOTOGRAPHER

Catharine's first child was born after a difficult pregnancy, and a weight gain of eighty pounds. At the time, she was a medical student, with a heavy schedule and stressful exams. Although her knowledge of nutrition should have helped her eat properly during this pregnancy, she had no time to cook and was never home. Of course, this had a direct effect on the quality of her Food-Qi, and the free flow of Qi in her body. When her child was born, Catharine realized that her diet had had a direct impact on her newborn child.

The baby, a beautiful girl, was born with cradle cap—scabs all over her head and behind her ears. "That's from all the pizza I ate . . . I ordered so much takeout during my pregnancy," Catharine told me. She was right. A course of baby probiotics to address the child's sugar imbalance and gentle massage with olive oil quickly took care of the cradle cap, but she resolved that her second baby would benefit from a better regime.

Both she and the second baby were the beneficiaries. Catharine's recovery from the first pregnancy had been long and complicated, because of the difficult circumstances. By the time she conceived her second child, Catharine was happily established in her professional practice. With the support of all her colleagues, she took excellent care of herself. She ate the right foods, adding wheat grass juice and excellent supplements to her diet. She had regular TCM treatments to balance her body. She was careful to get enough sleep and exercise. Her weight gain was healthy and adequate for the baby's needs but not excessive for herself.

This baby was born calm and problem-free, the very embodiment of the beauty of innocence. Within a month, Catharine began to feel her old self again. It helped that her mother came to provide her household with food, love and support. The little family had a regular routine, and she was allowed all the rest that she needed to rebuild her strength.

When Catharine brought her little newborn daughter into our clinic, we all jostled to take turns holding her. The baby was perfection itself. The small of her little neck was deliciously soft and fragrant; just holding her felt as if nourishing energy was pouring into each of us. No wonder she was so popular!

In my clinic, we begin to see babies with skin problems shortly after birth. From diaper rash to impetigo, eczema and psoriasis, little children suffer from a range of conditions that need treatment. I have been particularly struck with the frequency of these skin problems among adopted baby girls from China, aged from six months to two years. I think there must be an element of grief or sadness in these babies, many of whom have been abandoned or suffered before their adoptions. It is also possible that their biological mothers did not have proper nutrition during their pregnancies. Even if the orphanages where new parents pick up their children are terrible places, they may be the only home these babies have known, and the break from their caregivers there is another trauma.

I see many newly adopted Chinese girls, and most continue to come for treatment as they grow up. In general, by using a combination of herbs (both internally and topically); nutritional supplements, especially B vitamins, calcium, magnesium and cod liver oil; and tui na, we are able to stabilize these girls reasonably quickly.

We use the herbs to clear Heat and Dampness, cool the Blood, dispel Wind and elevate the babies' Qi. The supplements help to compensate for the poor diet during pregnancy and at the orphanage. The B vitamins are essential to promoting skin health. We teach the parents to massage their babies at home, and this makes a major difference in the balance and health of their bodies and spirits.

Skin is the vehicle of touch—we even like to touch ourselves! I really thought a lot about skin when I had my first baby: look at this perfect skin and touch it! I don't think I had ever felt anything that perfect before. I was fascinated with its perfection and smoothness. When you touch your own skin, it tells a story through marks and scars. I still have pebbles in my knee where the neighbour boy pushed me over in the driveway.

—BARBARA ASTMAN, ARTIST

One of my patients brought in just such a little girl shortly after her adoption. The new mother was very concerned: the child had constant nightmares. She was sleepless and always had a little chill directly to her Lung, leaving her with a chronic cough. The child had eczema on both elbows and knees. The mother trusted me as her physician, but she also wanted her child to have a continuing Chinese connection.

For a list of the most common skin conditions affecting babies, see page 91. The reference section includes recipes for topical herbal remedies and massage techniques, as babies cannot easily absorb remedies by mouth.

I was very moved by this little girl. As I treated her Lung Meridian, which is linked with sadness, I began to feel close to her, and I decided that I would indeed maintain a relationship with her. She is now seven years old, and I remain close to her.

I am very happy that my staff and I are able to help these Chinese baby girls become integrated into their new web of life, with healthy Qi and shining inner beauty. I will always have a special place in my heart for them.

ADOLESCENCE AND HEAVENLY WATER

A child's life is like a piece of paper on which
every passerby leaves a mark.
—*Chinese proverb*

As children grow older and begin to detach from their parents, they are forced to become more self-aware. The transition can be a rough ride for many adolescents; many are not comfortable in their own skins. My heart goes out to teenagers, both boys and girls. The nature of the changes between childhood and adulthood is often extreme, causing great upheaval in their lives, and for those around them.

Diana was just thirteen when I first met her. She had begun to experience her menstrual period, but it was irregular—in part because of her extreme thinness. Although she was an academic star with straight A+ marks and had a wonderfully supportive family, she suffered from a bloated Stomach, frequent indigestion and severe acne. Like her older siblings, also very successful in school, Diana was extremely focused—to the point that she had no social life beyond her family. Her beautiful face was covered with painful acne marks, but she suffered most from the uncontrolled and highly visible nature of the condition. When I first saw her, she sobbed as if her heart would break over this bodily rebellion against her perfect self-control.

I asked her if she loved herself. She said she did, and that was why she wanted to achieve success that would make her happy and please her parents. I explained to her that that was not self-love, which would require taking very good care of herself. The good news was that her body was signalling to her that it felt abandoned and unloved while it was still relatively easy to fix her health problems. If she were eating nutritiously, sleeping enough and getting healthy exercise, her Heavenly Water would flow easily and her Stomach problems would settle down.

Over the next six months, we undertook intense treatment for her acne, which gradually improved.

Diana had the good fortune of knowing herself well and feeling comfortable with her achievements. By working closely with me and taking her TCM treatments seriously, she was able to resolve her skin problems fairly easily. But many young women suffer from terrible self-esteem

For a description of the most common skin conditions affecting adolescents, see the reference section starting on page 77.

problems. These often manifest in the form of eating disorders, which are far more difficult to treat.

Marla is a good example of this heartbreaking phenomenon, which has become far too common in Western societies. The first time I saw her, she was so weak that her parents had to carry her into my clinic. She was reduced to skin and bones and had a tremor. She was fifteen. To my eyes, she looked as if she had a severe internal ailment of some kind, perhaps cancer.

Her parents told me they had just brought her out of the children's hospital two days before. Her diagnosis was anorexia nervosa—a disease I had never seen nor heard of in China. Learning that young women from well-to-do families who have access to good, healthy food are starving themselves came as a complete surprise to me at first, but it presents a recurring challenge, as I continue to see many such cases.

The way in which we relate to our bodies is very important in nurturing inner health and beauty. We are what we eat, and cutting off our food supply also cuts off our vital Qi. The resulting lack of nourishment leads inevitably to illness and deterioration.

I asked Marla why she did not want to eat, and she told me that in her mind, she saw herself as really fat. I tried to reconcile this with the tall, skeletal girl in front of me. Her skin was tight and dry to the touch. She was too dizzy to stand on her own. She had starved herself to the point of permanently damaging her small intestine, which had shrunk so that she could not keep food down, experiencing excruciating abdominal pain and vomiting. In my experience in China, patients who looked like her were either victims of starvation because there was no food available or dying of cancer.

Marla was extremely fearful. She trembled and cried out with pain at the slightest touch. I had to use short, ultra-fine needles to begin her acupuncture treatments. Her digestion was too fragile to handle with off-the-shelf herbal formulations.

Her parents patiently cooked herbs and made strong-smelling teas that Marla rejected at first. They spoon-fed her, trying again and again until she finally began to tolerate the treatment. Slowly, slowly, and with the support of a good psychotherapist, she began to regain her mental and physical strength, although some of the damage to her small intestine was irreversible—she will always have a slow digestive process, and it will take a very long time for her Qi to flow entirely freely.

The importance of friends and family in nurturing health and inner beauty cannot be exaggerated, but they are particularly vital during adolescence. Marla was very fortunate: she had two strong, loving, patient parents who were willing to go to incredible lengths to bring her to recovery, and she enjoyed unwavering support from the staff at Toronto's wonderful Hospital for Sick Children. This large and extended web of relationships, including many professionals and strangers supporting Marla and her parents, made a huge difference in the success of her treatment. Otherwise, she would likely have died.

The China in which I grew up was a world without psychotherapists. No one would have thought of looking to strangers for help with issues of the heart and mind. But friends and family were deeply engaged with one another and supported each other through life's difficulties. Although my own web of relationships is large and robust, the deep emotional connection among those closest to me remains the most important one in my life.

When I came to live in Canada, I was surprised by some of the differences in the way families interacted. For example, if a well-to-do family decided to give a car as a graduation present to a son or daughter, here is how the scene would likely unfold:

"We're proud of you, sweetheart. Here are the keys to your new car. Go and have a wonderful time with your friends!"

In a Chinese family, it would be more like this: "We are very proud of you. You have done a wonderful job. Now you are grown up enough to take responsibility for the whole family. Here are the keys to your new car. Granny will sit in the back with Mama, and Papa will sit up front with you. We can take a trip together under your leadership!"

Although my Western friends laugh when I tell them this story (and in fact, young Westerners might choose to forgo the new car rather than endure this scenario!), it does illustrate the strong bond within the Chinese family. To this day, my relationship with my family sustains me every day of my life. Because of my work, I see many illnesses and deaths among patients I care about deeply. However, when I learned that my sister was in critical condition, I was distraught: the fear of losing her was overwhelming.

I travelled to China to be by her side. The trip coincided with my fiftieth birthday. My other sister, my brother and I were constantly together, spending hours every day at the hospital with our ailing sibling. This privileged period of closeness and constant support for each other was filled with laughter and tears as we savoured our time together. I did what I could to contribute to my sister's treatment, along with the skilled physicians in the hospital. Slowly, she began to recover. This time with my family was the best birthday present I could have had.

As in the case of Marla's painful recovery, I see the difference that close family relationships and friendships make in a patient's healing. The web of support that we provide for each other reinforces the flow of vital energy among us, as well as the flow of Qi inside our bodies. We all need this.

FRIENDSHIP, 友谊 *(yǒu yì)*

> To meet an old friend in a distant country is like
> the delight of rain after a long drought.
> —*Chinese proverb*

When I first immigrated to Canada, I desperately missed my Chinese friends, who were so important in my life. I felt like a fish out of water. I wrote a letter every day to my friends in China. Whenever they got my letters, my friends would share them with each other, concerned about my well-being. Not being able to be with my friends was one of the most difficult aspects of adapting to a new country.

Imagine my surprise when I finally was able to plan a trip back to China to see my friends and this conversation ensued:

"Hey, I'm coming next week for a visit. I'm staying two weeks!"

Silence.

"Did you hear me?"

Silence . . . then, "Xiaolan, you shouldn't come."

"What?"

"Two weeks? Why are you doing something so foolish? It will take you twenty-four hours to get here and twenty-four hours to get home. Don't you realize how hard this will be on your body? It's better if you don't come."

Maybe I had already been in Canada too long at that point, but I was stunned. Didn't my friends want to see me? I missed them so much! And of course, that was also part of the problem: so many people would want to see me that the two-week trip would be no holiday at all. My friends believed that I was not respecting my body by undertaking such a brief, intense journey. They were also struck by how much living in the West had changed me.

My Chinese friends would hardly believe it if they saw how some of my Western patients live. Some of them think that their health and inner beauty will not be affected as they make major international trips several times a month and give themselves little or no time to recover and adjust. It was true that I had been influenced by living among them for so long.

In China, friends feel free to speak harsh truths to each other, but it is always because they are concerned about each other's health and well-being. What would be an act of friendship in China might be considered abominably rude and insensitive in Canada—and vice versa! My Canadian friends and patients do seem to forgive me for occasional brutal frankness in the clinic. They know it is my way of caring for them.

I am not alone in having had to learn to navigate trans-cultural issues as I made new friends in a new land. As I slowly began to acclimatize in my new country, I realized just how many others were in the same situation. Many of my patients had left their birthplaces to build a new life here. I took inspiration from their courage, and shared their journey, rebuilding a whole new web of relationships while treasuring the memory of those we had left behind.

I also had in common with so many immigrants the experience of leaving familiar work or a profession, and needing to adapt to a different, often inferior, station in life compared to what we had enjoyed back home. Many immigrant doctors become ultrasound or lab technicians or nurses because their original credentials are not recognized, or because they do not have Canadian experience. In addition to my TCM degree, I had been a Western-style surgeon in China. But to requalify to practise that part of my skill set in Canada would have delayed for years my ability to care for patients. I chose another path—not only because of the time I would have lost requalifying as a surgeon, but because I realized how little preventive medicine was available in the West. I had come to feel that I could make a much greater contribution as a TCM practitioner in this society.

Despite the frustrating process of overcoming the hurdle of credentials, Canada is a place that welcomes people from everywhere around the world. In China, I would never have had the opportunity to build close friendships with such a diverse range of people from so many different cultures. Eventually, Canada became my home and I am grateful to enjoy the new family of friends I have built over the years.

The mutual nurturing that comes from a community of friends is another important component to health and inner beauty. This became very clear through the experience of Hong, a newly immigrated Chinese patient referred to me by an oncologist. Hong was thirty-six. She had been in Canada for about six years with her husband and son, who was now seven years old. She had been diagnosed with Stage III breast cancer and was in shock—she had gone from diagnosis to mastectomy to radiation and chemotherapy in such a short time that she had barely had time to register what was happening to her.

I could understand how bereft she felt to be so far from her friends and family in China at such a difficult time. But Hong was fortunate. Her oncologist cared very much about her case, and was open to support from different branches of alternative medicine and to mitigating her side effects from chemotherapy.

But in addition to that, something unexpected then happened that touched Hong deeply: her entire neighbourhood mobilized to assist in her care. Her neighbours organized a schedule to cook for her, take her son to school and back, and free her husband to focus entirely on her care. Hong and her husband were astonished at the level of commitment their

For a description of the skin conditions affecting breast cancer patients, see page 95. The section includes recipes for herbal remedies for both topical and internal use.

neighbours demonstrated in helping them. In China, they might have expected such devotion from very close friends—but certainly not from neighbours who hardly knew them.

Today, Hong is in remission and is functioning very well. She has remained close to her neighbours and credits them with nourishing her into recovery and health. Friendship is a powerful and healing elixir. Hong radiates healthy Qi and inner beauty.

PERFECT UNION: COUPLES, SEX AND PARTNERSHIP, 完美结合 *(wánměi jiéhé)*

Married couples tell each other a thousand things without speech.
—*Chinese proverb*

A sexual union with a partner is the deepest, most intimate and satisfying relationship we can have: in TCM, it is the perfect union between Yin and Yang, the connection of the two fundamental energies that complete each other. While the traditional teachings speak only of man-woman partnerships, I have come to know many same-sex couples whose unions are every bit as genuine, life-affirming and deeply satisfying.

For the ancient Taoists, "clouds" represented the woman's Essence, her vaginal secretions, while "rain" represented the man's Essence, his semen. The man's fiery Yang energy heats up the woman's cool Yin energy in a natural interplay that mingles their bodily fluids and synchronizes their breathing in a perfect union. Neither energy dominates in this process: the cool, enduring Yin energy balances the short-lived, hot Yang energy.

Women absorb powerful Yang energy through sexual intercourse, while men receive the nurturing Yin energy to support their Yang. The act harmonizes water and fire. Men must excite women with their fire, while women, once warmed, take time to cool down. It makes sense that men are prone to falling asleep after expending their energy through ejaculation, whereas women are able to have multiple orgasms.

In ancient times, the Taoists believed that a man's semen was his Essence, or Jing. Wasting it in overly frequent ejaculations could deplete this vital Essence, accelerate the aging process and shorten his life. This is why men were encouraged to have sex regularly but to ejaculate only for procreation. The Taoists understood that the male orgasm and ejaculation are not one and the same. Few people today realize this, since they generally come so close together.

Surgeons who remove cancerous prostate glands often sever the nerve that governs erections in order to remove a safe margin of tissue. Sometimes, they can graft a nerve from another part of the man's body, but this is not always successful. Men who have had this surgery often feel diminished. But if they are fortunate enough to have good sexual intimacy with their partners, they often discover that no erection does not mean no orgasm—in fact, their orgasms can be more intense than ever before.

Similarly, women who have had hysterectomies must adjust to a different experience during sexual intercourse, and sometimes, uncomfortable vaginal dryness. True intimacy with a partner, supported by knowledge, can help a great deal. The balance of Yin and Yang energy between sexual partners, whether of the same or the opposite sex, can vary greatly. Each person has some of each type of energy, and sexual intimacy with a loving partner can circulate energy and stimulate the flow of Qi to the various parts of the body. This brings balance and healing, and as a bonus, it can slow the aging process.

The Taoists taught that retaining seminal fluid would increase a man's sexual capacity by increasing his vitality, as well as allowing him to bring his partner to orgasm so that he could absorb her Yin energy. Because women hold their orgasmic secretions within their bodies, they are not at the same risk of losing their vitality, and they are also able to absorb the Yang energy to strengthen them. Women were considered stronger, with a higher sexual capacity, greater sexual hunger and more sexual energy. After all, water can put out a fire!

For the Taoists, sexual intercourse was a means to replenish sexual energy and to ensure physical, emotional and mental well-being. They saw it as a spiritual experience, bringing together complementary opposites to unite with the larger universe of heaven and earth. Those whose sexual energy is depleted, or whose sexual needs are repressed, sometimes search for other sources of stimulation to fill the void, such as alcohol or drugs. This only weakens the mind and body, overactivating the senses and wasting precious Essence.

Women can feel that they are at once at their most vulnerable and at their most powerful during the sexual act. Making love attains its ideal between partners with a deep love and commitment for each other. But unfortunately, perfect union is not how many women experience sex. Many factors contribute to their dissatisfaction, perhaps above all the pressures of the culture and society that surround them.

When I was growing up in China in the 1970s, sex and relationships between men and women were heavily inhibited by judgmental attitudes, revealed by the Chinese proverb, "Runaway son, a shining jewel; runaway daughter, tarnished." Young people of the opposite sex did not feel free even to hold hands in public, and there was a stigma attached to merely showing interest in each other. Even in my early twenties, it was considered scandalous to be seen alone with a young man. Innocent friendships between boys and girls were impossible, and any contact between men and women was interpreted as a prelude to marriage within a short time.

A girl who defied these powerful social conventions was dirty and to be shunned. Many times a young woman tarred with this cruel brush—even though she was innocent—committed suicide rather than live with the disapproval of the society around her. One young woman, haunted by the consequences of being beautiful, disfigured her own face with acid in order to escape sexual harassment. Gossip was literally an agent of death.

A beautiful bird is the only kind we cage.
—*Chinese proverb*

This explains in part why I worked so hard to establish my credibility through my knowledge and skills. As a young Chinese woman, I hated even the concept that someone might find me beautiful. I did my best to hide my breasts under loose medical scrubs and made sure I was never alone with a person of the opposite sex.

As a young married woman, I had no idea what to expect. Like my friends at the time, I missed out on all of the potential of sexual activity to contribute to my health and well-being. I do not attribute the early failure of my marriage to this alone, but certainly the fact that I did not experience this deep and perfect union with my husband made it easier for me to leave him the year that my son was four years old.

I did have the example of an enduring union in my parents, who have been married since they were both seventeen years old. Their marriage was greatly tested by the storms of Chinese politics. At one point, my father was ordered to divorce my mother because of her political views. Because of his refusal to do so, he was transferred to another city and not allowed to see my mother for six years. During this time, we children only saw him for twelve days a year. This period was painful for my whole family.

Where thou art, that is home.

—EMILY DICKINSON, AMERICAN

POET (1830–1886)

Having survived these and many more challenges, my parents' enduring union has only become more perfect with age, resting on a bedrock of deep love and acceptance. My father is the living embodiment of acceptance and surrender, always giving credit to my mother and taking blame on himself. At the age of eighty-five, my mother is deeply in love with my father and will do anything for him.

When I think of inner beauty, the profound and complete acceptance and companionship between my parents is one of the first things that comes to my mind.

REFERENCE SECTION

TCM Techniques and Recipes for Preserving and
Building Your Inner Health and Beauty

Welcome to the reference section of *Inner Beauty*. After I had written my first book, *Reflections of the Moon on Water*, I found that everywhere I went, people asked for very practical advice on how to live according to the principles of TCM, and how to take care of their own health and that of their loved ones through the techniques and remedies it has to offer. Rather than try to convey technical information in the text of this book, I decided that including a reference section would provide it for those who seek it, without interrupting the narrative flow for those who simply want to read the stories and philosophy of health and inner beauty.

Because of my ongoing desire to reach out to Western practitioners and work together in the best interests of our patients, I asked Dr. Sandy Skotnicki to comment on those cases where we have worked together, or where it is enlightening to consider the similarities and differences in our approaches to specific conditions. These comments and exchanges between us are marked 对话 (duì huà), which is Mandarin for "dialogue."

I know that not all my readers live in centres where TCM practitioners are easily accessible, so I have given thought to ways in which they can gain access to the ingredients and treatments that are the most useful for the broad range of conditions we are addressing in this book—conditions as disparate as rosacea and yeast infections. I have addressed the needs of adults, children and babies, so that the entire family can have access to TCM healing.

Because babies cannot usually tolerate herbal preparations by mouth, I have provided baby massage techniques that will help parents address blockages in the Qi and stimulate the baby's Meridians to promote health and well-being. These techniques are demonstrated in pictures throughout the reference section. The dots on the pictures show the relevant massage points. Massage the baby on these points using a clockwise circular motion and firm pressure, but not enough to make the baby uncomfortable. For points on the back, work from the top down. You may use oil, lotion or aloe gel. Sesame oil, olive oil, coconut oil, sweet almond oil or Purple Rejuvenation Massage Oil (see recipe on page 188) are all suitable for baby massage. Babies love to be massaged, and you will quickly find that the experience is healing and bonding for both of you.

This reference section is organized by condition and topic, concentrating on skin and hair, the most obvious "messengers" of your state of inner health and beauty. Where I have included recipes for herbal preparations, I have named the ingredients in English but have also included the pharmaceutical names for the herbs, as well as their names in Chinese characters and the romanized Pinyin, which guides the reader on pronunciation. I have used the same approach in the glossary, which begins on page 212. My thinking here is that this approach will maximize the chances that the reader can purchase the herbs from a Chinese herbalist anywhere in the world while reducing the risk of errors or misunderstanding. Most towns and cities have at least one Chinese herbalist or TCM practitioner. Even if he or she does not speak English, if you bring this book, you should have no trouble obtaining what you need.

Please note that it is important not to cook herbs in metal pots. Use ceramic, enamel or glass suitable for stove-top cooking.

For the moment, I will not be recommending any particular online suppliers, but my website, www.chinesehealing.ca, contains a question-and-answer section to which you may submit your queries. In future, if I am able to research the quality and reliability of specific suppliers, I will feel free to recommend them to readers and patients.

A

ACNE, 粉刺 (fěn cì)

The first thing anyone sees when they look at someone is their face. When the facial skin is hot and inflamed, covered with acne, it is very difficult for that person—no matter how calm and self-confident—to feel beautiful. And indeed, a body that is generating enough Heat at the surface of the skin to produce acne is not in balance.

Acne can be triggered by hormonal or other imbalances in the body, as a result of the onset of Heavenly Water, Ripening the Fruit or high stress. Treating it may require different approaches at different points in the patient's life cycle. In general, TCM seeks to regulate menstruation in women with acne, and the digestive system in men with the condition. We can use external treatments and acupuncture to disperse and eliminate lesions and to speed up healing time.

You may find that adult acne and acne rosacea (which are described below) flare up around the mouth during pregnancy (Ripening the Fruit) as a result of changes in hormone levels. These problems tend to be purely temporary. It is important to know that many of the drugs normally used for these conditions are unsafe for use during pregnancy. Aside from a topical cream, I do not treat this condition during pregnancy, as I do not feel that any of the internal remedies I have are safe during pregnancy.

My friend Dr. Sandy Skotnicki also prefers not to use any medication during Ripening the Fruit, especially in the first trimester, when the fetal brain is developing. She says, "We do have a few options for pregnant women with acne after the first trimester: topical erythromycin, metronidazole, azelaic acid and glycolic acid peels. Glycolic acid is based on sugar cane and is very helpful for treating acne in pregnant and breastfeeding women."

ADULT ACNE, 成人痤疮 (chéng rén cuó chuāng)

In adolescents, acne tends to be a result of hormonal upheaval. When acne returns in adulthood, it is more likely to be the result of other factors such as stress and metabolic problems such as overactive sebaceous glands. Adult acne can produce painful and deep cysts, with a risk of scarring. It is no easier psychologically for adult patients than for adolescents, as the pressure to be presentable and attractive, both in the workplace and in their personal lives, never lets up.

TCM Treatment

Three Yellow Cooling Wash

When the skin is very inflamed, we make a herbal infusion known as the "three yellow" formula and use it to wash the lesions twice a day.

1 L	water
20 g	amur cork tree bark (*Cx. Phellodendri*, 黄柏, huáng bǎi)
20 g	Chinese rhubarb (*Rx. et Rz. Rhei*, 大黄, dà huáng)
15 g	Baikal skullcap (*Rx. Scutellariae*, 黄芩, huáng qín)
15 g	sophora root (*Rx. Sophora*, 苦参, kǔ shēn)

In a ceramic, enamel or glass saucepan, bring the water to a boil. Add all the herbs and simmer until the liquid is reduced by half. Chill for at least 20 minutes before using. Store in the refrigerator.

Three Cooling Face Masks

With acne, the face is often hot. Here are three examples of soothing, cooling face masks for topical use. Each should be chilled for at least 20 minutes before applying and refrigerated when not in use. Apply them interchangeably, once a day, after using the Three Yellow Cooling Wash. Leave the mask on for 20 minutes, then wash off gently with clear, lukewarm water.

Herbal Face Mask

- 1 egg white
- 5 g talcum powder (*Talcum*, 滑石粉, huá shí fěn)
- 5 g dahurian angelica powder (*Rx. Angelica dahurica*, 白 芷粉, bái zhǐ fěn)
- 5 g Chinese ground orchid powder (*Rz. Bletilla*, 白芨粉, bái jī fěn)
- 3 g Chinese rhubarb root powder (*Rx. et Rz. Rhei*, 大黄粉, dà huáng fěn)
- 1 g borneol powder (*Dryobalanops aromatica or Blumea balsamifera*, 冰片粉, bīng piàn fěn)

Combine all the ingredients to make a paste. Refrigerate for 20 minutes before applying to face.

Fruit Face Mask

- 1 apple
- Juice of half a lemon
- 3 drops lavender essential oil

In a food processor, purée together the apple, lemon juice and lavender essential oil. Refrigerate for 20 minutes before applying to face.

Vegetable Face Mask

For this recipe, if you can't find bitter melon, the juice of half an English cucumber will do. Use an electric or hand-cranked juicer to obtain the juices.

- 125 mL soft tofu
- Juice of 1 celery stalk
- Juice of ¼ bitter melon (*Mormordica charantia*, 苦瓜, kǔ guā)

Combine tofu, celery juice and bitter melon juice to make a paste. Refrigerate for 20 minutes before applying to face.

Antibacterial Face Mask
Apply this mask once a day for 20 minutes, then rinse gently with clear, lukewarm water.

- 10 g burnt gypsum fibrosum powder (*Gypsum fibrosum*, 烧石膏粉, shāo shí gāo fěn)
- 10 g calcitum powder (*Calcitum*, 寒水石粉, hán shuǐ shí fěn)
- 5 g Baikal skullcap powder (*Rx. Scutellariae*, 黄芩粉, huáng qín fěn)
- 5 g gallnut powder (*Rhus chinensis*, 五倍子粉, wǔ bèi zǐ fěn)
- 1 g borneol powder (*Dryobalanops aromatica* or *Blumea balsamifera*, 冰片粉, bīng piàn fěn)
  Boiled water

Combine together all the powders with enough boiled water to make a paste. Refrigerate for at least 20 minutes before using.

Jade Skin Tea
Drink 500 mL of this tea per day, 250 mL in the morning and 250 mL in the evening. There is no need to refrigerate this tea.

- 15 g Chinese foxglove (raw) (*Rx. Rehmannia recens*, 生地黄, shēng dì huáng)
- 15 g hawthorn fruit (*Fr. Crataegi*, 山楂, shān zhā)
- 15 g trichosanthes root (*Rx. Trichosanthes*, 天花, tiān huā)
- 15 g hedyotis (*Hb. Oldenlandia*, 白花蛇舌草, bái huā shé shé cǎo)
- 12 g ningpo figwort (*Rx. Scrophuloriae*, 玄参, xuán shēn)
- 12 g dwarf lily-turf, or Japanese snake's beard (*Ophiopogon Japanicus*, 麦冬, mài dōng)

10 g Baikal skullcap (*Rx. Scutellariae*, 黄芩, huáng qín)

10 g Chinese lobelia (*Hb. Lobeliae*, 半边莲, bàn biān lián)

10 g barbed skullcap (*Rx. Scutellariae barbata*, 半枝莲, bàn zhī lián)

2 L water

In a ceramic, enamel or glass saucepan, combine all the ingredients. Let soak for 20 minutes to half an hour, then bring to a boil and simmer for 40 minutes, or until the liquid is reduced to 500 mL.

Silky Skin Maintenance Wash
Once the inflammation is under control, wash the lesions every other day with this wash to help maintain the skin in good condition.

100 g dried mung beans (*Phaseolus mungo*, 绿豆, lǜ dòu)

1.25 L filtered water

100 g grated fresh daikon radish (*Raphanus sativus*, 萝卜, luó bo)

Place the mung beans in a bowl and cover with cold water. Let them soak overnight, then drain them, reserving the mung beans. Bring the filtered water to a boil and add the reserved mung beans and daikon. Simmer for 45 minutes. Drain, reserving the liquid. Discard the pulp. Store the reserved liquid in the refrigerator.

Full Moon Jade Tea
Drink 250 mL of this tea in the morning and 250 mL in the evening. There is no need to refrigerate the tea.

15 g sophora root (*Rx. Sophora*, 苦参, kǔ shēn)

15 g amur cork tree bark (*Cx. Phellodendri*, 黄柏, huáng bǎi)

15g trichosanthes root (*Rx. Trichosanthes*, 天花, tiān huā)

10 g Baikal skullcap (*Rx. Scutellariae*, 黄芩, huáng qín)

10 g Chinese rhubarb (*Rx. et Rz. Rhei*, 大黄, dà huáng)

2 L water

In a ceramic, enamel or glass saucepan, combine all the ingredients. Let soak for 2 hours, then bring to a boil and simmer for 40 minutes, or until reduced to 500 mL.

对话 (duì huà)

Sandy: In adult women, especially if the acne is on the lower half of the face, I investigate their hormonal situation: Are they on oral contraceptives? Do they get a premenstrual flare of the condition? Are their menstrual cycles regular? Any of these factors can trigger adult acne. For some women, going on oral contraception will resolve the issue, although this may be controversial in patients over the age of thirty-five. Spironolactone is a mild and very effective medication that slightly changes testosterone levels and clears adult acne within a couple of months in some cases.

In women who are trying to get pregnant or who cannot or prefer not to undertake hormonal therapies, intense pulsed light (IPL), which is a phototherapy, is a good option.

Xiaolan, I know we agree that adult acne is becoming more common and that it seems to be related to stress and hormone levels in women. But our approaches are different: I treat it with targeted hormone therapy and you treat it holistically.

Xiaolan: TCM also believes that diet plays an important role in generating the Heat and the Dampness that manifest as acne. I do think that we should explore whether we can obtain better outcomes by collaborating. It seems to me that this is an example of an area where TCM and Western medicine can be complementary.

What You Can Do for Acne (Lifestyle Changes)

Cut down on fatty and sweet foods and eat more fruits and vegetables. Do not squeeze the lesions when the skin is very inflamed, especially in the triangle below the nose, in the lower part of the face ("the golden triangle"). The veins in this area lack the protective "gates" that slow the progress of infection everywhere else in the body. In extreme cases, squeezing acne lesions in this area can cause a rush of Toxins to the brain.

ACNE ROSACEA, 痤疮酒渣鼻 (cuó chuāng jiǔ zhā bí)

Rosacea is a chronic inflammatory condition that is most common in middle-aged people but which can also affect young adults and the elderly. It starts as redness and visibly dilated capillaries on the forehead, cheeks, nose and chin and around the eyes. Later on, small red bumps (papules) and pus-filled bumps (pustules) can appear, but not the blackheads and whiteheads typical of other forms of acne.

Rosacea can be provoked or aggravated by emotional factors, digestive or endocrine dysfunction, alcohol or excessive caffeine use, overindulgence in spicy foods, or exposure to sun and heat. It is more common among people who flush easily, for example, when they eat spicy food or when they are embarrassed. While rosacea is more common in women than in men, chronic and deep inflammation of the nose (chronic rhinophyma, or "drinker's nose") is more common in men than in women.

Sometimes the eyes are affected (ocular rosacea). This involves the oil gland above the eye and damages the lubricant function of the tears, thereby causing eye irritation that can become chronic.

TCM Treatment

Soothing Rosacea Herbal Wash

Wash the affected areas morning and evening with this preparation.

- 15 g   barbed skullcap (*Rx. Scutellariae barbata,* 半枝莲, bàn zhī lián)
- 15 g   hedyotis (*Hb. Oldenlandia,* 白花蛇舌草, bái huā shé shé cǎo)
- 15 g   gardenia (*Fructus Gardeniae jasminoidis,* 栀子, zhī zi)
- 15 g   trichosanthes root (*Rx. Trichosanthes,* 天花, tiān huā)

15 g   Baikal skullcap (*Rx. Scutellariae*, 黄芩, huáng qín)

1 L   water

In a ceramic, enamel or glass saucepan, combine all the ingredients. Let soak for 2 hours, then bring to a boil and simmer for 45 minutes. Pour through a sieve, reserving the liquid. Discard the pulp. Chill the reserved liquid for at least 20 minutes before using. Store in the refrigerator.

Soothing Rosacea Treatment Powder

Apply this powder to affected areas once a day.

50 g   puncture vine powder (*Fr. Tribulus terrestris*,白蒺藜粉, bái jílí fěn)

25 g   seeds of Job's tears, or coix powder (*Se. Coicis*, 薏苡仁粉, yì yǐ rén fěn)

25 g   ground oyster shells (*Concha ostrea*, 牡蛎粉, mǔ lì fěn)

Combine the seeds of Job's tears and puncture vine powder. Add the ground oyster shells and stir to combine. Store in a sealed jar at room temperature.

Herbal Face Mask for Rosacea

Apply this mask to affected areas once a day for two weeks. Leave it on for 20 minutes, then rinse gently with clear, lukewarm water.

30 g   wild chrysanthemum powder (*Fl. Chrysanthemi indici*, 野菊花粉, yě jú huā fěn)

20 g   burnt alum powder (*Potassium Aluminum Sulphate*, 烧明矾粉, shāo míng fán fěn)

20 g   Chinese rhubarb root powder (*Rx. et Rz. Rhei*, 大黄粉, dà huáng fěn)

10 g   sulphur powder (硫黄粉, liú huáng fěn)

10 drops peppermint oil (*Hb. Menthae*, 薄荷油, bò he yóu)

Combine all the ingredients with enough water to make a paste. Refrigerate for at least 20 minutes before using. Store in the refrigerator.

Nourishing Rosacea Vegetable Face Mask
Apply this mask once a day, leaving it on for 20 minutes. Rinse gently with clear, lukewarm water.

1/2	cucumber, peeled
25 mL	aloe gel, or a 10- to 13-cm piece of aloe
25 mL	raw honey (*Mel*, 生蜂蜜, shēng fēng mì)

In a food processor, purée all the ingredients together. Chill for at least 20 minutes before using. Store in the refrigerator.

对话 (duì huà)

Sandy: I tailor the treatment to the degree to which the acne rosacea bothers the patient. Cosmetically, when a patient's skin turns very red because of broken or blocked capillaries, IPL phototherapy or Vbeam laser treatments can be very effective ways to restore some normality to their skin colour. I would also use prescription medications such as metronidazole and azelaic acid to combat inflammation. For more serious cases, I will add oral antibiotics, principally tetracycline, doxycycline and minocycline. For very severe cases that recur after discontinuing the antibiotic, I will suggest isotretinoin (Accutane).

Some rosacea patients flush easily and so markedly that they find it debilitating. For these patients, we use medications that block the nervous control of flushing, most commonly beta blockers.

In mild cases with only low levels of redness, I might recommend that they use sunscreen and avoid red wine and hot, spicy foods, and for some patients, dairy products.

Xiaolan: Body Heat comes from the Liver and the Stomach and rises through the central Meridians. Rosacea patients have very acidic bodies. You'll find that many of them are sensitive to orange juice and other acidic foods. I ask them to watch their diets and not drink alcohol, which is linked to the Stomach Meridian.

Sandy: My thinking on this continues to evolve, but it's now clear to me that inflammatory foods also play a role. The backbone of rosacea treatment for me is a combination of topical and oral medications. But when I have a patient who is allergic to those medications, I feel pretty much handcuffed.

Xiaolan: Those cases would probably benefit from a TCM approach, Sandy!

What You Can Do for Acne Rosacea
Avoid hot and spicy foods, smoking and alcohol. Avoid secondary infection of the nose through good hygiene. Wash the face with lukewarm water and make sure to dry your skin before applying topical medication.

ALLERGIES, 过敏 (guò mǐn)

Allergies—at least type I allergies, which are what most people associate with the word—are very common. Some people are hypersensitive to substances that are harmless to most people. In some cases, the sensitivity is so acute it can be fatal. When a person is exposed to the offending substance, an antibody known as immunoglobulin E (IgE) activates the white blood cells known as mast cells and basophils into an extreme inflammatory response. Hives, hay fever and asthma are all common examples of allergic reactions.

Mild allergies are relatively easy to manage, causing symptoms such as allergic conjunctivitis (eye infections), itchiness and a runny nose. But extreme allergies may result in anaphylactic reactions.

Anaphylaxis can present many symptoms, as histamines are released throughout the body. The reactions can develop very quickly, over a few minutes, or take several hours. The most common areas affected are the skin (in 80 to 90 per cent of cases, including symptoms such as generalized hives, itchiness, flushing, and swelling of the lips, tongue or throat, which can be life-threatening); the respiratory system (in 70 per cent of cases, including symptoms such as shortness of breath, wheezing and lack of oxygen); the gastrointestinal system (in 30 to 45 per cent of cases, including symptoms such as cramps, abdominal pain, diarrhea and vomiting); the heart and vascular system (in 10 to 45 per cent of cases, including symptoms such as coronary artery spasm, with subsequent myocardial infarction or dysrhythmia); and the central nervous system (in 10 to 15 per cent of cases, including symptoms such as fainting, loss of bladder control and muscle tone, anxiety and panic).

Anaphylaxis can happen in response to any type of allergy, including allergies to insect bites or stings, foods, medication and latex rubber. The most common food allergies are to peanuts, tree nuts, shellfish, fish, milk and eggs.

TCM Treatment
Make and use the Three Yellow Cooling Wash as described on page 80, adding a small bunch of fresh coriander (*Coriandrum sativum*, 香菜, xiāng cài) and three slices of fresh ginger root (*Rz. Zingiberis*, 生姜根, shēng jiāng gēn) to the recipe.

对话 (duì huà)
Sandy: Type I allergic reactions, like the ones discussed above, are treated by allergists, not dermatologists. The first line of defence is avoidance of the allergen, but there are various medications available, such as antihistamines, when the substance causing the problem cannot be avoided (for example, in ragweed season). Poison ivy

typically causes a type IV allergic reaction. I tell patients that while the plant's oils cause a skin rash, it's likely they could eat the plant (not that they should!) without serious harmful consequences. The adage in Western medicine is "once allergic, always allergic."

Xiaolan: In TCM, there are many kinds of allergies that can be reversed as we balance Kidney Qi. Of course, I would not attempt this in a child who is severely allergic to peanuts, for example. But in many patients, a process of detoxification and healing can remove the body's reaction to certain foods and substances.

Sandy: My mind has been opened on this subject, both through discussions with you, Xiaolan, and through evolving research in Western medicine on allergy reversals and vaccination. This is definitely another area for collaboration.

ALOPECIA AREATA

See Hair Loss, page 124.

ANDROGENETIC HAIR LOSS (Thinning)

See under Hair Loss, page 132.

B

BABIES

Baby skin is so important in protecting little ones from Toxins and illnesses both in the here and now and also throughout their whole lives. Their skin is far thinner and more delicate than adult skin—and we sense this when we caress its silky softness. When a baby is clean, healthy and balanced, this delicate skin glows and subtly gives off one of the loveliest smells imaginable.

In this reference section, the conditions affecting babies, TCM treatments, recipes and dialogues with Dr. Sandy Skotnicki are organized by condition in alphabetical order: Cheilitis, Diaper Rash, Intertrigo, Infantile Seborrheic Eczema (listed under Eczema), Infectious Eczematous Dermatitis, Measles, and Oral Candidiasis or Thrush (listed under Thrush).

Baby Massage for Overall Health

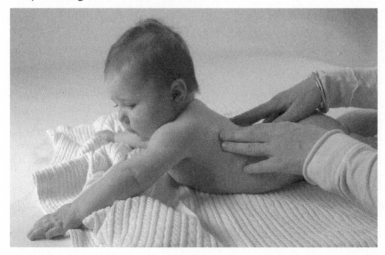

BASAL CELL CARCINOMA
See Skin Cancer, page 171.

BINGE DRINKING, 酗酒 (xù jiǔ)
TCM Treatment

To treat skin affected by heavy drinking, see the treatments given for acne rosacea on pages 85 to 87. To cleanse the liver, prepare the following infusion.

Liver Cleanse Tea

Drink 250 mL of this tea in the morning and 250 mL in the evening for 7 to 14 days. There is no need to refrigerate the tea.

20 g	seeds of Job's tears, or coix (*Se. Coicis*, 薏苡仁, yì yǐ rén)
15 g	root bark of shaggy-fruited dittany (*Cs. Dictamni*, 白鲜皮, bái xiān pí)
15 g	plantain (*Hb. Plantaginis*, 车前草, chē qián cǎo)
15 g	akebia caulis (*Cs. Akebia*, 木通, mù tōng)
12 g	bupleurum (*Rx. Bupleuri*, 柴胡, chái hú)
12 g	Chinese gentian (*Rx. Gentiana*, 龙胆草, lóng dǎn cǎo)
10 g	alisma (*Rz. Alismatic*, 泽泻, zé xiè)
3 g	licorice (*Rx. Glycyrrhizae*, 甘草, gān cǎo)
2 L	water

In a ceramic, enamel or glass saucepan, combine all the ingredients. Let soak for 2 hours, then bring to a boil and simmer for 40 minutes, or until liquid is reduced to 500 mL.

对话 (duì huà)

Sandy: Some of the systemic medications I prescribe are absolutely incompatible with the use of alcohol. And yet, among some patients with severe cases of disease, alcohol may provide relief from stress and pain that is considerable. I find that those who follow my instructions to stop their alcohol consumption during the therapy achieve significant improvements. I have no way of establishing whether or not abstinence from alcohol is a key factor in their recovery.

What You Can Do for Binge Drinking

If alcohol consumption is part of your life, you should pace yourself and use it sparingly. Try drinking a full glass of water for every glass of wine or alcohol to dilute it, to counter its dehydrating effect, and to give your liver a chance to process it at normal speed, rather than accumulating it as a Toxin. Your liver needs an hour to process one regular glass of wine, a beer or a mixed drink.

BREASTFEEDING: Sore, Cracked Nipples, 疼痛, 乳头破解 (téng tòng, rǔ tóu pò jiě)

Although people who do not know any better might assume that breastfeeding is a simple, natural procedure, it can be surprisingly difficult for some first-time mothers to find the right technique. The surest sign that a lactating mother needs help with technique is sore, cracked nipples.

If the baby is sucking only on the nipple, rather than on the whole areola, with a wide open mouth and tongue down, the baby will suck too hard in an attempt to get more milk. The milk sinuses that deliver the liquid are in the areola and need to be compressed by the baby's mouth in order to work smoothly. It is also important for mothers to release the baby's suction before removing the child from the breast. Unfortunately, mothers with sore, cracked nipples sometimes give up breastfeeding, believing that there is something wrong with their milk supply. They should see a professional lactation consultant, who can help evaluate the problem and provide coaching.

Sore, cracked nipples may also result when babies have anky-loglossia (tongue-tie), because they may not be able to latch on to the areola properly. A baby with a candida infection (thrush) can spread it to the mother's nipples, causing redness, tenderness and a burning sensation.

Women with moderate to severe nipple pain, cracks, fissures, ulcers or a discharge from the nipples may have a bacterial infection (most often *Staphylococcus aureus*), which may delay the healing process.

TCM Treatment

Soothing Licorice-Orchid Paste

This paste is soothing for sore or infected breasts. If the breasts are red and hot, be sure to refrigerate it for 20 minutes before use. Do clean the paste from the nipple before breastfeeding, although it is not harmful to the baby.

50 g	Chinese ground orchid powder (*Rz. Bletilla*, 白芨, bái jī)
30 g	licorice powder (*Rx. Glycyrrhizae*, 甘草粉, gān cǎo fěn)
100 mL	glycerine (*Symphytum officinalis*, 甘油, gān yóu)

Combine all the ingredients to form a paste. Store at room temperature, and apply to nipples as needed.

Cooling Antibacterial Healing Paste

Apply this paste to the breasts as needed. Clean the paste from the nipples before nursing.

30 g	Chinese honey locust spine powder (*Sp. Gleditsiae*, 皂角刺粉, zào jiǎo cì fěn)
30 g	trichosanthes root powder (*Rx. Trichosanthis*, 天花粉, tiān huā fěn—literally "heavenly flower powder")
20 g	Chinese arborvitae twig and leaf powder (*Cacumen Biotae orientalis*, 侧柏叶粉, cè bó yè fěn)

20 g   Chinese rhubarb root powder (*Rx. et Rz. Rhei,* 大黄粉, dà huáng fěn)

20 g   peppermint powder (*Hb. Menthae,* 薄荷粉, bò he fěn)

20 g   honeysuckle flower powder (*Fl. Lonicera,* 金银花粉, jīn yín huā fěn)

Combine all the ingredients with enough water to make a paste. Store in the refrigerator.

What You Can Do for Sore, Cracked Nipples

Wash the nipples with warm water and rub some of your own milk on them. Breast milk is sterile and therapeutic. If the nipples are cracked, avoid the use of nipple shields, which can promote bacterial growth. If the problem persists, it is likely because of the way the baby is latching on to the breast and requires help from a professional lactation consultant.

If the problem develops into fever and redness of the breast, then it is mastitis and involves blocked ducts. Unblocking them is best done with a pump to express milk, although this is painful. Warm and hot compresses and massaging the breasts can help, and breastfeeding should be continued as much as possible.

BREASTS: Pain and Illness, 乳房护理 (rǔ fáng hù lǐ)

For Radiodermatitis, see page 165; for Chemotherapy, see page 101.

At my clinic, I see a great many women with breast cancer, not only because the disease is tragically common, but also because many women with this disease are seeking alternative solutions. Most of these patients have already had surgery, radiation or chemotherapy, or some combination of these treatments. They feel that they have tried everything, and think of us as their last hope to return to health.

Any cancer is a wake-up call, but breast cancer attacks women in a place that is central to their identity, both as mothers and as sexual beings. Many women feel a profound sense of betrayal—and even anger—when their bodies "let them down" in this way. In TCM, there is a direct link between anger, resentment and other strong emotions, through the path of the Liver Meridian, to the breasts. It is logical to assume that retained anger and other strong emotions can play a role in triggering this devastating disease. I discussed this subject more extensively in my first book, *Reflections of the Moon on Water*. Here, we will look more closely at the impact of breast cancer and its treatments on a woman's skin.

Paget's disease is a primary breast cancer that presents in the skin as chronic inflammation and crusting of the nipple. It begins below the surface and rises to the surface. It is not metastatic.

There are four different skin patterns of metastatic breast cancer, which can remain localized. They are

- sclerodermatous (hard, tethered areas of skin that do not move well);
- telangiectatic (reddish patches where there is a loss of feeling);
- erysipeloid (the skin is red and looks like orange peel because the cancer has gone into the dermis); and
- nodular (red bumps on the skin).

POST-SURGERY SCAR TISSUE, 手术后的疤痕组织
(shǒushù hòu de bāhén zǔzhī)

All surgery is traumatic to some extent. But breast cancer surgery is among the most difficult because of the dramatic change to a woman's appearance and sense of herself. The amount of resulting scar tissue will depend upon whether the surgery is a small lumpectomy or a radical mastectomy. In addition to the removal of breast tissue, the patient must manage a drain for a number of days afterwards, which is both unpleasant and painful. If the surgery involves the loss of lymph glands, as it often does, there will be additional conse-quences, such as swelling and post-operative vulnerability to infec-tion in the areas where the lymphatic drainage is affected.

It is important to trust our bodies, which can often help us develop new ways to work around trauma and loss, and also provide the sup-port that the body needs to heal and to learn these new ways.

TCM Treatment

Whole Earth Massage Oil

Use this oil to massage both the scar tissue and the areas where lymph glands have been removed. This will help the body find new pathways for lymphatic drainage.

30 g	bushy knotweed (*Rx. Polygoni cuspidati*, 虎杖, hǔ zhàng—literally "tiger's cane")
30 g	amur cork tree bark (*Cx. Phellodendri*, 黄柏, huáng bò or huáng bǎi)
30 g	Baikal skullcap (*Rx. Scutellariae*, 黄芩, huáng qín)
15 g	poppy capsule (*Per. Papaveris somniferi*, 罂粟壳, yīngsù ké)
15 g	schisandra fruit (*Fr. Schisandra chinensis*, 五味子, wǔ wèi zǐ)
15 g	garden burnet root (*Rx. Sanguisorbia*, 地榆, dì yú)
10 g	borneol powder (*Dryobalanops aromatica* or *Blumea balsamifera*, 冰片, bīng piàn)
250 mL	sesame oil (*Sesamum*, 麻油, má yóu)
	Egg-Yolk Oil (see recipe on page 186)

In a ceramic, enamel or glass saucepan, combine all the ingredi-ents except Egg-Yolk Oil, and cook until the herbs become dark yellow. Remove from the heat and pour through a sieve, reserving the oil mixture. Discard the herbs. Combine the reserved oil mix-ture with the Egg-Yolk Oil.

对话 (duì huà)

Sandy: I suggest scar massage with silicone gel or silicone sheets. If the patient is very bothered by the scar, we can do fractional laser treatments to diminish its visibility.

Xiaolan: That would work well with my treatment: local acupuncture with small needles.

C

CALCIUM DEFICIENCY
Bone Soup

Our bodies always need calcium, but there are times when we need more than usual to be in balance, healthy and feeling beautiful. This soup is excellent for women who are Ripening the Fruit, as it helps to prevent cramps, as well as to form the baby's teeth and bones. It is also very useful at other times of life when our bodies need lots of calcium—for example, it can help to prevent hair loss in both men and women.

    1 kg   beef, pork or chicken bones
    2.5 L   cold water
    25 mL   apple cider vinegar

Place the bones in a large pot. Add the cold water and apple cider vinegar. Bring to a boil. Cover and reduce the heat; simmer for 4 hours.
Makes 6 servings.

CHEILITIS, 唇炎 (chún yán) or 唇风 (chún fēng—literally "lip wind")

Cheilitis is an inflammation of the mucous tissues of the mouth that is most common among children and young women. It can be either acute or chronic and can be triggered by exposure to sun and wind, by constant licking or biting of the lips, or by allergies to substances in products such as flavouring agents or other chemicals in lipstick, sunscreen, toothpaste, dental floss or mouthwash or even on the mouthpieces of musical instruments. Cheilitis generally starts as redness and swelling that proceeds to dryness and scales that peel off and form scabs repeatedly. There may be burning pain.

TCM Treatment

Soothing Lip Wash

Use this to wash the lips three times a day for as long as needed.

30 g	mung beans (*Phaseolus mungo*, 绿豆, lǜ dòu)
15 g	dandelion (*Hb. Tara*, 蒲公英, pú gōng yīng)
10 g	pagoda tree flower (*Rx. Sophora*, 槐花, huái huā)
10 g	purslane (*Portulaca oleracea*, 马齿苋, mǎ chǐ xiàn)
10 g	green tea (*Camellia sinensis*, 绿茶, lǜ chá)
1.5 L	water

In a ceramic, enamel or glass saucepan, combine all the ingredients. Let soak for 2 hours, then bring to a boil and simmer for 20 minutes. Pour the mixture through a sieve, reserving the liquid. Discard the pulp. Refrigerate the reserved liquid for 20 minutes before using. Store in the refrigerator.

If this condition arises in a baby, parents may also massage the child.

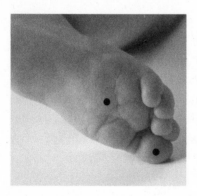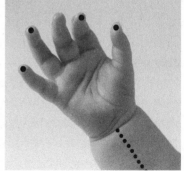

对话 (duì huà)

Sandy: If the lips do not settle down, we will treat the inflammation with a corticosteroid. Once it is calmed, we reintroduce products one at a time, one per week, avoiding flavouring agents, particularly mint-based ones. If there is still a problem, we proceed to patch-test for allergens, starting with the most common agents used in lip and dental care products.

What You Can Do for Cheilitis

Avoid substances that irritate the lips, or potential allergens such as alcohol, cigarettes, lipstick and rich and spicy food. Don't lick, bite or pick at your lips. In terms of cosmetics and products, less is more. Refrain from using all potential irritants and allergens except baking soda to brush your teeth, unflavoured dental floss and a petrolatum-based barrier cream to keep your lips moist.

CHEMOTHERAPY, 化疗 (huà liáo)

Cancer is unique in that it is the only disease where we try to cure the body by poisoning it. This is why chemotherapy can be so painful as our bodies struggle with Toxins designed to kill the cancer tissues. Aside from general fatigue, nausea and other side effects of chemotherapy, the skin is a prime area of activity in the body's efforts to rid itself of these Toxins. This is why we see rashes, mouth ulcers, hair loss and many other conditions that result directly or indirectly from chemotherapy treatments.

In our clinic, we see many patients who develop skin, nail and mouth conditions as a result of chemotherapy, and our treatments are designed to support these patients as they undergo it.

TCM Treatment

Soothing Fruit and Mineral Bath

Sit in this bath for 20 minutes.

40 g   Chinese rhubarb (*Rx. et Rz. Rhei*, 大黄, dà huáng)

30 g   mirabilite, or Glauber's salt (*Mirabilitum*, 芒硝, máng xiāo)

30 g   sophora root (*Rx. Sophora*, 苦参, kǔ shēn)

30 g   mume fruit (*Fr. Prunus mume*, 乌梅, wū méi)

10 g   burnt alum (*Potassium Aluminum Sulphate*, 烧明矾, shāo míng fán)

1 L   water

In a ceramic, enamel or glass saucepan, combine all the ingredients. Let soak for 2 hours, then bring to a boil and simmer for 45 minutes. Pour into a warm bath.

Calming Bark and Mineral Paste

Use this topical paste as needed, applying it to irritated skin.

100 g   burnt gypsum fibrosum powder (*Gypsum fibrosum*, 烧石膏粉, shāo shí gāo fěn)

100 g   talcum powder (*Talcum*, 滑石粉, huá shí fěn)

30 g   indigo root powder (*Rx. Indigo naturalis*, 青黛 粉, qīng dài fěn)

30 g   amur cork tree bark powder (*Cx. Phellodendri*, 黄柏 粉, huáng bǎi fěn)

15 g   smithsonite or calamine (*Smithsonitum*, 炉甘石, lú gān shí)

5 g   borneol powder (*Dryobalanops aromatica or Blumea balsamifera*, 冰片, bīng piàn)

         Sesame oil (*Sesamum*, 麻油, má yóu)

Combine all the powders with enough sesame oil to make a paste. Store at room temperature.

Healing Herb and Vegetable Tea

This tea should be drunk twice, once in the morning and once in the evening, but for the second time, use 500 mL of water and reduce it to 250 mL.

- 50 g   Chinese yam (*Rx. Dioscorea*, 山药, shān yào)
- 20 g   adzuki bean (*Phaseolus angularis*, 赤小豆, chì xiǎo dòu)
- 20 g   seeds of Job's tears, or coix (*Se. Coicis*, 薏苡仁, yì yǐ rén)
- 20 g   cicada slough (*Per. Cicadae*, 蝉蜕, chán tuì)
- 20 g   lotus seed (*Se. Nelumbinis*, 莲子, lián zǐ)
- 15 g   astragalus (*Rx. Astragali*, 黄芪, huáng qí)
- 12 g   Chinese black dates (*Fr. Jujubae*, 大枣, dà zǎo)
- 1 L   water

In a ceramic, enamel or glass saucepan, combine all the ingredients. Soak for half an hour. Bring to a boil, then simmer for 45 minutes, or until reduced to 250 mL.

CHICKEN POX
See *Varicella Zoster, page 198.*

CHLOASMA
See *Melasma, page 145.*

CORNS AND CALLUSES, 鸡眼和胼胝 (jī yǎn hé pián zhī)
Corns and calluses are the skin's way of protecting itself from excessive pressure and friction from improper footwear. While, in many cases, removing the source of the problem will make it go away, corns and calluses can also turn into more serious problems, especially among diabetics or others with circulatory problems.

TCM considers corns and calluses to be manifestations of Blood stasis, cutting off nourishment to the skin.

TCM Treatment

Ginger Citrus Foot Bath

Soak your feet in water and trim the corns or calluses a bit. Then make this solution and use it while it is still very warm, soaking your feet in it for 20 minutes once a day.

- 50 g grated fresh ginger root (*Rz. Zingiberis*, 生姜根, shēng jiāng gēn)
- 30 g belvedere fruit (*Fr. Kochia*, 地肤子, dì fū zǐ)
- 20 g tangerine peel (*Citrus reticulata*, 陈皮, chén pí)
- 10 g safflower flower or carthamus (*Fl. Carthemi*, 红花, hóng huā)
- 2 L   water

In a large ceramic, enamel or glass saucepan, combine all the ingredients. Let soak for 2 hours, then bring to a boil and simmer for 20 minutes.

Peachy Soft Foot Paste

Apply this paste to affected areas once a day. It will soften corns and calluses. This recipe will make enough to last a few weeks, depending on usage.

- 50 g peach kernel powder (*Se. Persica*, 桃仁粉, táo rén fěn)
- 50 g skin of wolfberry root or lycium bark powder (*Rx. Lycium chinensis*, 地骨皮粉, dì gǔ pí fěn)
- 10 g safflower flower or carthamus powder (*Fl. Carthemi*, 红花粉, hóng huā fěn)
        Sesame oil (*Sesamum*, 麻油, má yóu)

Combine all the powders with enough sesame oil to make a paste. Store in a sealed jar at room temperature.

对话 (duì huà)

Sandy: Calluses are there for a reason: to protect vulnerable skin from friction, often from inappropriate footwear. It is important to keep calluses under control before they turn into corns, which are more painful and more difficult to manage. Unfortunately, patients are sometimes resistant to addressing the cause of the problem—especially if it means getting rid of their favourite stiletto heels.

Xiaolan: It certainly seems to be very difficult to convince women that shoes that damage their feet do not make them more beautiful.

Sandy: Unfortunately, the price is steep, but it is paid many years after the behaviour that caused it. That does make it tough to change the behaviour.

In the meantime, the first course of action is to pare down the excess skin with a surgical blade. Medicated pads containing salicylic acid can do the same thing gradually. As we age, the architecture of the feet can also change: arches fall, there is less protective fatty tissue, and bones become more prominent. Podiatrists can fit patients with orthotics that can help under these circumstances.

CRADLE CAP

See Infantile Seborrheic Eczema, page 119.

D

DERMATITIS
ALLERGIC CONTACT DERMATITIS, 过敏性接触性皮炎 (guò mǐn xìng jiē chù xìng pí yán) or 漆疮 (qī chuāng— literally "lacquer sore")

TCM refers to allergic contact dermatitis as "lacquer sores" because early practitioners would often see it in people who worked with lacquer, a Toxic substance that is acrid and hot. This can stir Wind and generate Fire, attack the skin and interstices (cou li), constrain the Liver channel and spread to the skin, causing inflammation, swelling, redness and rashes. The disease can range from acute to chronic, but it is always provoked by contact with an allergen of some kind.

Reactions to allergens are highly individual. One person can touch a substance and be completely unaffected; another can touch it without a problem for years, then develop an allergy. Contact allergy results from repeated exposures, in a process known as sensitization. Once the person is sensitized, exposure to the substance will elicit a repeat reaction, sometimes worsening or spreading over time. Your immune system has a memory, and reactions are specific to each exact substance. For example, exposure to airborne particles of lacquer or some other allergen can cause itchy skin and swelling, most visible in areas with loose skin, such as the eyelids and the scrotum. There can be a rash that turns into blisters that rupture and form yellow crusts, and may spread. Once someone is sensitized to an allergen, it is almost impossible to reverse this.

In the adult years, parents find themselves working hard to raise children and manage a household. Their hands are often in soapy water, solvents, cleaning fluids and other chemicals that can cause allergic contact dermatitis. Even if you are very busy, it is important to address these discomforts, as they have a way of deteriorating into more serious problems, as well as draining energy from your body and pleasure from your life.

Babies and young children can also experience allergic contact dermatitis. Parents can use the baby massage techniques below.

TCM Treatment

Land and Sea Soothing Wash

Wash the affected areas with this solution twice a day.

50 g	red carrots (*Daucus carota* var. *sativa*, 红胡萝卜, hóng hú luó bo)
50 g	coriander (*Coriandrum sativum*, 香菜, xiāng cài)
50 g	water chestnuts (*Eleocharis dulcis*, 马蹄, mǎ tí)
50 g	seaweed (*Hb. Sargassii*, 海藻, hǎi zǎo)
50 g	glabrous greenbrier root (*Rz. Smilacis glabrae*, 土茯苓, tǔ fú ling)
20 g	cicada slough (*Per. Cicadae*, 蜕蝉, chán tuì)
2.5 L	water

In a large ceramic, enamel or glass saucepan, combine all the ingredients. Let soak for 2 hours, then bring to a boil and simmer for 15 minutes. Pour through a sieve, reserving the liquid. Discard the pulp. Store the reserved liquid in the refrigerator.

Soothing Root and Mineral Paste

Apply this paste to lesions twice a day.

50 g	burnt alum powder (*Potassium Aluminum Sulphate*, 烧明矾粉, shāo míng fán fěn)
30 g	garden burnet root powder (*Rx. Sanguisorbia*, 地榆粉, dì yú fěn)
30 g	sophora powder (*Rx. Sophora*, 苦参粉, kǔ shēn fěn)
30 g	honeysuckle flower powder (*Fl. Lonicera*, 金银花粉, jīn yín huā fěn)

30 g Chinese rhubarb root powder (*Rx. et Rz. Rhei,* 大黄粉,
dà huáng fěn)
Sesame oil (*Sesamum,* 麻油, má yóu)

Combine all the powders with enough sesame oil to make a paste.
Store the paste in the refrigerator.

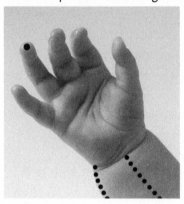 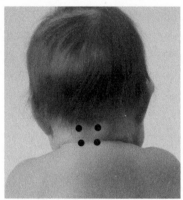

对话 (duì huà)

Xiaolan: Sandy, this is one of those conditions where I feel that
your services are very helpful—particularly to identify which allergens are causing the problem.

Sandy: We never used to see allergic contact dermatitis in children,
but we are seeing more of it now—probably because of the vast
increase in the number of ingredients that we find in products that
are used on the skin. We are a long way from the old days when
mothers used only plain white soap, baby oil and petroleum jelly
on their babies. Today, there are entire aisles in the drugstore filled
with various scented and specialized preparations that really are
not necessary for little ones, for whom less is truly more. Parents
are often reassured by words like "hypoallergenic" or "for sensitive
skin," but in fact these descriptions do not come with any legal
requirements, and in my experience they do not mean much.

We can only identify the allergens causing the problem through allergy patch testing. Once the allergen is identified, avoidance is the only treatment. If the allergen remains unidentified or the skin develops eczema, we treat it with hydrocortisone.

What You Can Do for Allergic Contact Dermatitis
If the area is red, swollen or weeping, avoid contact with hot water, do not scratch and avoid spicy or irritating food. If you suspect it is a reaction to a topical product, see a dermatologist and consider having patch testing done. Once you discover where the problem is coming from, avoid contact with known allergens. If you or your child has a history of contact dermatitis, you should take this into account when planning travel, work or exposure.

INFECTIOUS ECZEMATOUS DERMATITIS, 传染性湿疹样皮炎 (chuán rǎn xìng shī zhěn yàng pí yán) or 湿毒疮 (shī dú chuāng—literally "Damp Toxin sore")
Infectious eczematous dermatitis is difficult to distinguish from contact dermatitis, especially in the first stages. It presents as a moderate to severely itchy scaling or oozing eruption, often caused by a bacteria such as staphylococcus. The lesions may spread with scratching. Severe cases may induce fever, swelling of nearby lymph glands and a spike in white blood count. The disease can be provoked or aggravated by an irregular diet (including too much tea, alcohol, seafood and spicy food), emotional stress, a rash or having an impatient nature or being irritable and restless. A chronic phase can cause long-term damage to Yin and consumption of Blood, which leads to Dryness.

TCM Treatment
Slow-Down Bath
Prepare this bath and soak the body in it for 20 minutes.

50 g   sophora (*Rx. Sophora*, 苦参, kǔ shēn)

50 g   shaggy-fruited dittany (*Cs. Dictamni*, 白鲜皮, bái xiān pí)

50 g   wild chrysanthemum (*Fl. Chrysanthemi indici*, 野菊花, yě jú huā)

40 g   catmint *(Hb. Schizonepeta*, 荆芥, jīng jiè)

30 g   gallnut (*Rhus chinensis*, 五倍子, wǔ bèi zǐ)

5 L   water

In a large ceramic, enamel or glass saucepan, combine all the ingredients. Let soak for 2 hours, then bring to a boil and simmer for 45 minutes. Pour through a sieve, reserving the liquid. Discard the pulp. Pour the reserved liquid into a bath, adding enough water to cover the body.

Precious Yellow Diamond Calming Paste

This wonderful paste calms itching and reduces inflammation, Heat and pain. Apply it to the affected areas as needed. The paste does not need to be refrigerated, but if the skin is very hot and itchy, chilling it may help.

50 g   powdered seeds of Job's tears, or coix (*Se. Coicis*, 薏苡仁 粉, yì yǐ rén fěn)

50 g   gypsum fibrosum powder (*Gypsum fibrosum*, 石膏粉, shí gāo fěn)

30 g   hedyotis powder (*Hedyotis diffusa*, 白花蛇舌草粉, bái huā shé shé cǎo fěn)

30 g   Baikal skullcap powder (*Rx. Scutellariae*, 黄芩 粉, huáng qín fěn)

20 g   sulphur (硫黄 粉, liú huáng fěn)

Sesame oil (*Sesamum*, 麻油, má yóu)

Combine all the powders with enough sesame oil to make a paste.

Tui na will also help this condition, especially in babies.

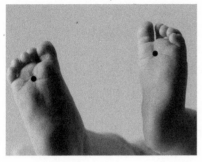 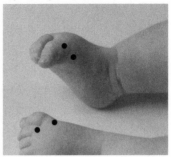

对话 (duì huà)

Sandy: I think I do a good job of getting acute conditions like these under control. I generally mix an antibacterial with a corticosteroid to get rid of the bacterial infection or irritating colonization and bring the inflammation down. In some cases, oral antibiotics are needed, because corticosteroids will not work on infected skin.

Xiaolan: My treatments are intended to soothe and balance to prevent recurrence, but your approach works more quickly for acute cases, Sandy.

Sandy: Bacteria love inflamed skin. So a person with chronic dermatitis who scratches and breaks the protective skin barrier becomes a prime candidate for infected eczema. This bacterial infection becomes an overlay to the original problem and makes treating the problem more complex—which is where you come in!

What You Can Do for Infectious Eczematoid Dermatitis

Avoid fish, shellfish, spicy food, alcohol, coffee or strong tea during treatment. Do not scratch or wash the lesions with hot water, to avoid secondary infection. Any infectious process requires prompt treatment: see your doctor right away.

DIAPER RASH, 尿布疹 (niào bù zhěn) or 臀部淹没疮 (tún bù yān mò chuāng—literally "buttock-submerging sore")

Babies can suffer a great deal when their soft, vulnerable skin spends many hours a day in contact with wet diapers. If a dirty diaper often smells like ammonia, this is because the irritant actually forms in a chemical reaction between stools and urine. In TCM, this foul stuff is considered to be turbid Damp-Heat that attacks the skin. When the baby is not changed promptly (this can happen not only through neglect but also simply through a long sleep), skin lesions can develop in the area covered by the diaper. It starts with moist, glazed areas with defined borders and progresses from there to erosion and ulceration. Sometimes, secondary infections follow, caused by a strain of yeast called *Candida albicans*, characterized by pustules. Diaper rash is a form of contact dermatitis, and we look for it on convex surfaces—the places where the baby's skin has been in contact with the diaper. In the folds, we are more likely to find intertrigo (see page 140); pustules are the telltale sign of candida infection. If the rash proceeds to infection, the baby will feel burning heat and stabbing pain will have fever and constipation. The tongue will be red with a scant coating, and the pulse will be rapid.

Babies suffering from diaper rash can be restless and may cry from the pain and discomfort. They may also develop a fever and lose their appetite. While modern super-absorbent disposable diapers have reduced the occurrence of diaper rash, the renewed interest in cloth diapers can reverse this progress, unless they are carefully washed in very hot water and properly dried. If this is not done systematically, the diapers can retain Fire pathogens, which can combine with Wind and Heat to cause skin irritations.

Faithful use of Gold and Purple Massage Oil (*Rx. Lithospermum*, 紫草根油, zǐ cǎo gēn yóu—see recipe on page 165), will usually

prevent diaper rash altogether. However, if it does occur, we concentrate on topical treatments, such as bathing the baby in
Licorice-Chrysanthemum Water (*Rx. Glycyrrhizae*, 甘草菊花水,
gān cǎo jú huā shuǐ) and then applying Green Velvet Calming
Baby Bottom Paste. If the baby's condition is severe, we use
Green Satin Baby Bottom Cooling and Nourishing Paste. (See
recipes below.)

Licorice-Chrysanthemum Water (*Rx. Glycyrrhizae*, 甘草菊花水, gān
cǎo jú huā shuǐ)

  20 g   chrysanthemum (*Fl. Chrysanthemi indici*, 菊花, jú huā)
  10 g   licorice (*Glycyrrhizae preparata*, 甘草, gān cǎo)
  15 g   amur cork tree bark (*Cx. Phellodendri*, 黄柏, huáng bò
         or huáng bǎi)
   2L   water

Combine the herbs with water and soak for half an hour. Bring
to a boil, then simmer for 45 minutes. Filter the water and use
it to wash the baby's bottom. The water can be kept at room
temperature.

Green Velvet Calming Baby Bottom Paste
Apply this paste to the baby's bottom as needed.

  45 mL   mung bean powder (*Phaseolus mungo*, 绿豆粉, lǜ dòu
          fěn)
          Olive oil (*Olea europaea*, 橄榄油, gǎn lǎn yóu)

Combine the mung bean powder with enough olive oil to form a
paste. Store in a sealed jar at room temperature.

Green Satin Baby Bottom Cooling and Nourishing Paste
Apply this paste to the baby's bottom as needed.

  75 mL   peppermint powder (*Hb. Menthae*, 薄荷 粉, bò he fěn)

1 mL   borneol powder (*Dryobalanops aromatica* or *Blumea balsamifera*, 冰片粉, bīng piàn fěn)
Raw honey (*Mel*, 蜂蜜, fēng mì)

Combine the peppermint powder and borneol powder with enough honey to make a paste. Store in a sealed jar at room temperature.

Parents can also massage their baby to prevent and treat diaper rash.

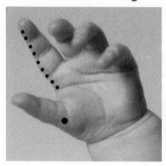 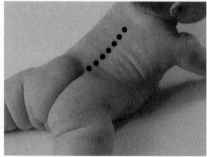

对话 (duì huà)

Sandy: Xiaolan, this is one of the areas where Western doctors recognize the possibility that there can be dietary triggers to a condition. I often advise parents to cut back on acidic juices, for example, if an older baby has diaper rash—or at least to cut juices with water. For the rest, it seems to me that common sense is in order here: soothe the irritation and create a barrier from the irritant. I like to recommend a barrier agent such as Ihle's Paste, an old-fashioned zinc oxide cream, applied in a thick layer, to keep the skin dry and protected. If we suspect a candidal infection, we will prescribe an antifungal medication, such as clotrimazole, in a corticosteroid cream, followed by the barrier cream.

DRY SKIN PROBLEMS

See Xerosis, page 207.

E

ECZEMA, 湿疹 (shī zhěn)

There are many different sub-types of eczema, and it differs somewhat at different ages. The types more typical among babies and children are described separately below.

Among older people, there are three sub-types that occur more commonly: asteatotic eczema (also called eczema craquelé), where the skin gets so dry it cracks; stasis eczema on the lower legs, which results from blood pooling in the veins as circulation slows down with age; and nummular eczema, which is coin-shaped dry, inflamed patches on the legs. This latter condition can arise in younger age groups for genetic reasons, but most of these conditions arise because of the natural aridity and slower renewal cycles of aging skin. Atopic eczema typically improves with age.

In TCM, we first establish what is causing the eczema and dispel the problem factors. There may be Exterior Causes settling in the skin, such as Wind (resulting in multiple lesions and pronounced itching), Dampness (resulting in lower body sores that do not heal) or Heat (resulting in red and swollen skin, possibly leading to infections by Toxins); or there may be Interior Causes involving the Heart (resulting in red, inflamed and extremely itchy skin), Spleen (resulting in maceration, where the skin turns white from wetness and becomes vulnerable to fungal infections or erosion) or Kidney (which can lead to Kidney Yin or Kidney Yang deficiencies). These internal problems can move out to the skin and interstices (腠李, còu lǐ). Dietary irregularities can also lead to a depletion of Yin liquids and binding of Damp-Heat. In TCM, eczema is also known as 史真 (shǐ zhēn, meaning

"Damp eruption"), 峰石床 (fēng shí chuáng, meaning "Wind-Damp sore") or 金银闯 (jīn yín chuǎng, meaning "wet spreading sore").

TCM Treatment

Crackling Skin Bath

Soak in this tub for 20 minutes.

50 g	cnidium (*Se. Cnidium*, 蛇床子, shé chuáng zǐ)
50 g	belvedere fruit (*Fr. Kochia*, 地肤子, dì fū zǐ)
30 g	Chinese rhubarb (*Rx. et Rz. Rhei*, 大黄, dà huáng)
30 g	Baikal skullcap (*Rx. Scutellariae*, 黄芩, huáng qín)
30 g	amur cork tree bark (*Cx. Phellodendri*, 黄柏, huáng bò or huáng bǎi)
30 g	stemona root (*Rx. Stemona*, 百部, bǎi bù)
5 L	water

In a large ceramic, enamel or glass saucepan, combine all the ingredients. Let soak for 2 hours, then bring to a boil and simmer for 45 minutes. Pour through a sieve, reserving the liquid. Discard the pulp. Add the reserved liquid to a warm bath with enough water to cover the body.

Soothing Azure Anti-itch Powder

Apply this powder to the lesions three times a day.

50 g	gypsum fibrosum powder (*Gypsum Fibrosum*, 石膏粉, shí gāo fěn)
30 g	talcum powder (*Talcum*, 滑石粉, huá shí fěn)
15 g	indigo root powder (*Rx. Indigo naturalis*, 青黛粉, qīng dài fěn)
10 g	burnt alum powder (*Potassium Aluminum Sulphate*, 烧明矾粉, shāo míng fán fěn)
5 g	borneol powder (*Dryobalanops aromatica* or *Blumea balsamifera*, 冰片粉, bīng piàn fěn)

5 g calomel powder (*Calomelas,* 轻 粉, qīng fěn)

Combine all the ingredients and store in a sealed jar.

Fragrant Herbal Healing Mask for Eczema

If the face is affected with eczema, use this mask or Cooling Watermelon Rind Cream (see recipe below). Apply this mask to affected areas once a day. Leave it on for 20 minutes, then rinse gently with clear, lukewarm water.

15 g gromwell root powder (*Rx. Lithospermum,* 紫草粉, zǐ cǎo fěn)

10 g skin of wolfberry root or lycium bark powder (*Rx. Lycium chinensis,* 地骨皮粉, dì gǔ pí fěn)

10 g powdered cloves (*Fl. Carylphylli,* 丁香粉, dīng xiāng fěn)

10 g angelica root powder (*Rx. Angelica sinensis,* 当归粉, dāng guī fěn)

Almond oil

Combine all the powders with enough almond oil to make a paste. Store in a tightly covered container. It does not require refrigeration.

Cooling Watermelon Rind Cream

Apply this cream to affected areas once a day. Leave it on for 20 minutes, then rinse gently with clear, lukewarm water. If the eczema is all over your body, you will need a whole watermelon. For smaller areas, reduce the quantities in the same 3:1 proportion of water-melon to yogurt as below.

1 watermelon

Plain whole-milk yogurt

Scoop out the white part of the rind of a watermelon and place in a food processor. Add yogurt in a 3:1 ratio (for 750 mL watermelon, add 250 mL yogurt), and purée until combined. Keep refrigerated.

Herbal Rainbow Eczema Tea
Drink 250 mL of this tea in the morning and 250 mL in the evening. This tea does not need to be refrigerated.

15 g	catmint *(Hb. Schizonepeta,* 荆芥, jīng jiè)
15 g	dandelion (*Hb. Tara,* 蒲公英, pú gōng yīng)
15 g	honeysuckle flower (*Fl. Lonicera,* 金银花, jīn yín huā)
15 g	forsythia fruit (*Fr. Forsythia,* 连翘, lián qiáo)
12 g	*Saposhnikovia divaricata* root (*Rx. Ledebouriella,* 防风, fáng fēng)
12 g	Yedeon's violet or viola (*Hb. cum Radice Violae yedoensitis,* 紫花地丁, zǐ huā dì dīng)
12 g	prunella (*Spica prunellae,* 夏枯草, xià kū cǎo)
12 g	capillaries (*Artemisia capillaris,* 茵陈, yīn chén)
3 g	licorice (*Rx. Glycyrrhizae,* 甘草, gān cǎo)
2 L	water

In a ceramic, enamel or glass saucepan, combine all the ingredients. Let soak for 2 hours. Bring to a boil and simmer for 40 minutes, or until reduced to 500 mL.

对话 (duì huà)

Sandy: We encourage older patients to be especially conscientious about moisturizing their skin. This is often enough to prevent the eczema. Genetic forms of eczema such as atopic dermatitis and seborrheic dermatitis can still occur despite preventive measures, although they can be mitigated somewhat. In many of my patients, stopping the use of a range of irritating cleansing products and detergents is enough to vastly improve their condition without the use of additional medication.

What You Can Do for Eczema

Patients should avoid washing with hot water, soap and detergents. They should also avoid consuming fish, shellfish, spicy food and alcohol.

INFANTILE SEBORRHEIC ECZEMA, 婴儿脂溢性皮炎 (yīng ér zhī yì xìng pí yán) and CRADLE CAP, 摇篮帽 (yáo lán mào)

Seborrheic dermatitis is common and chronic throughout life. To a certain extent, in babies it is related to the mother's diet and state of health during both pregnancy and breastfeeding. Newborn infants are most likely to suffer from infantile seborrheic eczema. You will see it as moist, defined areas of redness in the folds of the skin at the groin or the neck. It is mildly itchy.

When it occurs on the scalp, it may also present as greyish yellow or brownish yellow oily scales that can cover all or part of the scalp, a condition known as cradle cap. TCM recognizes that if a mother eats too much fatty, sweet, spicy or fried food, fish or seafood during pregnancy and while breastfeeding, this will impair the transportation capacity of her Spleen and generate Damp-Heat.

The same will apply to children who have the same dietary habits. A mother can pass Heat Toxins and turbid substances in the Blood to her baby through breastfeeding. Plump babies tend to suffer more from excess Dampness, while thin and weak babies are more vulnerable to excess Heat. Where the Damp-Heat accumulates over a long period, this can result in chronic disease. While it is not common in young children, seborrheic dermatitis often starts up at puberty, when new hormones trigger the release of sebum.

TCM Treatment

The principle of the treatment is to clear Heat and cool the Blood, transforming the Dampness, relieving Toxicity and pain. With babies, it is very important to bring the condition under control as soon as possible. To treat cradle cap, wash the area with Gentle Softening Cradle Cap Wash (see recipe below).

Gentle Softening Cradle Cap Wash
Use this preparation to wash the baby's head twice a day.

15 g   licorice (*Rx. Glycyrrhizae,* 甘草, gān cǎo)
15 g   wild chrysanthemum (*Fl. Chrysanthemi indici,* 野菊花, yě jú huā)
1.5 L   water

In a ceramic, enamel or glass saucepan, combine all the ingredients. Let soak for 2 hours, then bring to a boil and simmer for 20 minutes. Pour through a sieve, reserving the liquid. Discard the pulp. After washing the baby's head with the liquid, apply Bitter Golden Balancing Paste (see recipe below).

Bitter Golden Balancing Paste
Apply this paste twice a day after washing the affected area with the Gentle Softening Cradle Cap Wash (see recipe above).

20 g   goldenseal powder, or Chinese goldthread root (*Rz. Coptidis,* 黄连根粉, huáng lián gēn fěn)
        Rice vinegar (good quality)

Combine goldenseal powder with enough rice vinegar to make a paste. Store in a sealed jar.

Healing Mother's Milk Tea
If the condition is severe, the breastfeeding mother should drink 500 mL of this infusion per day. The tea does not need to be refrigerated.

15 g   mat rush (*Juncus effusus,* 灯心草, dēng xīn cǎo)
15 g   honeysuckle flower (*Fl. Lonicera,* 金银花, jīn yín huā)

15 g   rice sprouts (*Orzya sativa*, 谷芽, gǔ yá)

15 g   licorice (*Rx. Glycyrrhizae*, 甘草, gān cǎo)

12 g   lophatherum (bamboo leaves) (*Lophatherum gracile Brongniart*, 淡竹叶, dàn zhú yè),

12 g   root bark of shaggy-fruited dittany (*Cs. Dictamni*, 白鲜皮, bái xiān pí)

12 g   plantain (*Hb. Plantaginis*, 车前草, chē qián cǎo)

1.5 L   water

In a ceramic, enamel or glass saucepan, combine all the ingredients. Let soak for 2 hours, then bring to a boil and simmer for 20 minutes. Pour through a sieve, reserving the liquid. Discard the pulp.

Black Balancing Antibacterial Paste

If the baby's condition is severe, apply this paste to the scalp twice a day. Leave on for 20 minutes, then rinse gently with clear, luke-warm water.

30 g   gypsum fibrosum powder (*Gypsum fibrosum*, 石膏粉, shí gāo fěn)

20 g   amur cork tree bark powder (*Cx. Phellodendri*, 黄柏粉, huáng bǎi fěn)

10 g   burnt alum (*Potassium Aluminum Sulphate Dodecahydrate*, 烧明矾粉, shāo míng fán fěn)

10 g   indigo root powder (*Rx. Indigo naturalis*, 青黛 粉, qīng dài fěn)

        Vegetable oil

Combine all the herbs with enough vegetable oil to make a paste. Store in a sealed jar.

In the case of a baby, parents can perform this massage.

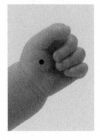 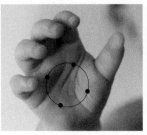 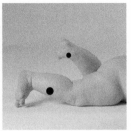

对话 (duì huà)

Sandy: Xiaolan, I don't know if you have the same experience, but I find that parents are often almost as disturbed by the fact that this condition affects the baby's appearance as by the discomfort that it can cause.

Xiaolan: Health and beauty go hand in hand! If the baby's body is balanced, this condition will not appear.

Sandy: It will go away without treatment, but most parents prefer to treat it. We recommend mineral oil, almond oil or olive oil to treat cradle cap, covering it overnight and washing the next day, over a period of time. If the child is scratching and aggravating the condition, we use a corticosteroid lotion to relieve it.

What You Can Do for Infantile Seborrheic Eczema

Avoid fatty, sweet, spicy or fried food, fish and seafood while pregnant or breastfeeding. It is important to soften the dry scales with some kind of oil, and to keep the scalp clean to prevent secondary infection.

EXANTHEM SUBITUM

See Roseola, on page 166.

F

FUNGAL INFECTIONS, 真菌 (zhēn jūn) and YEAST INFECTIONS, 酵母感染 (jiào mǔ gǎn rǎn)

Most fungi are not toxic or dangerous to humans. Nature is full of fungi, such as mushrooms and the benign fungi that reside permanently on the skin. Only a very few fungi are likely to live on humans, feeding on dead keratin (protein) cells in the top layer of the skin, hair and nails. If they are able to burrow in deeper, for example, in people with weakened immune systems, fungal infections can become chronic, very damaging and difficult to cure, but this is very rare.

Generally, fungi that are transmitted from animals to humans cause more severe inflammations than those that are transmitted from person to person.

See also Yeast Infections, page 210.

H

HAIR LOSS, 脱发 (tuō fà)

Both men and women associate their hair very closely with their looks and are very self-conscious about hair loss, even when it is very minor. Few of us realize that at any one time, only 90 per cent of our hair is growing normally, while 10 per cent of it is in a resting phase. Every two to three months, the resting hairs fall out so that new hair can take their place. During pregnancy, the rise in estrogen in our bodies promotes hair growth and reduces hair loss. This change in the hair's regular cycle can delay the loss of the "resting" hairs so that it happens all at once later. Almost half of all women experience excessive shedding of hair one to five months after pregnancy. This delayed hair loss usually peaks three to four months after delivery, as the hair follicles rejuvenate themselves. Hair loss returns to normal rates within six to twelve months.

Sometimes, abnormal hair loss during hormonal changes (Ripening the Fruit, stopping oral contraceptives or other hormone therapies, miscarriage or stillbirth, abortion or a hormonal imbalance) can be due to vitamin or mineral deficiencies.

TCM Treatment for Postpartum Hair Loss

TCM associates hair with the Blood; excessive hair loss after pregnancy is a sign that the Blood needs replenishing after so much has gone into making and delivering the baby.

Postpartum Fruit and Flower Root Wash

Use this wash once a day for 10 days. Do not use shampoo during this time.

30 g	fresh ginger root (*Rz. Zingiberis*, 生姜根, shēng jiāng gēn)
20 g	fleeceflower root (*Rx. Polygori multiflori*, 何首乌, hé shǒu wū)
20 g	psoralea fruit (*Fr. Psoralea*, 补骨脂, bǔ gǔ zhī)
15 g	Chinese arborvitae twig and leaf (*Cacumen Biotae orientalis*, 侧柏叶, cè bó yè)
1.5 L	water

In a ceramic, enamel or glass saucepan, combine all the ingredients. Let soak for 2 hours, then bring to a boil and simmer for 30 minutes. Pour through a sieve, reserving the liquid. Discard the pulp. Apply liquid to the hair. Wrap the head in a towel and leave the solution on for one hour. Rinse the hair with clear water.

Happy Growth Tea

Drink 250 mL of this tea in the morning and 250 mL in the evening for 15 days, then take 15 days off. Repeat this cycle twice more. The tea does not need to be refrigerated.

20 g	cinnamon bark (*Cx. Cinnamomi*, 肉桂, ròu guì)
20 g	astragalus (*Rx. Astragali*, 黄芪, huáng qí)
15 g	angelica root (*Rx. Angelica sinensis*, 当归, dāng guī)
15 g	Chinese foxglove root cooked in wine (*Rx. Rehmanniae conquitae*, 熟地黄, shú dì huáng)
15 g	poria (*Poria*, 茯苓, fú líng)
12 g	Szechuan lovage root (*Rz. Ligustici Wall.*, 川芎, chuān xiōng)
12 g	white peony root (*Rx. Paeonia alba*, 白芍, bái sháo)
12 g	codonopsis (*Rx. Codonopsitis*, 党参, dǎng shēn)
12 g	white atractylode root (*Rx. Atractylodes alba*, 白术, bái zhú)
6 g	honey-fried licorice (*Rx. Glycyrrhizae preparata*, 炙甘草, zhì gān cǎo)
2 L	water

In a ceramic, enamel or glass saucepan, combine all the ingredients. Let soak for 2 hours, then bring to a boil and simmer for 40 minutes, or until reduced to 500 mL.

对话 (duì huà)
Sandy: This condition is also called telogen effluvium, and it is quite common. For most patients in my practice, it is enough to reassure them that their hair will come back before too long. However, in some patients, low iron levels caused by bleeding, stress or other reasons can turn the condition from acute to chronic. In these women, I would increase their dietary iron. If they have finished breastfeeding, I might also recommend minoxidil, a medication that can increase the blood supply to the hair follicles and reactivate growth. I do not believe that any of the shampoos and topical products that are on the market will help.

Xiaolan: As you can see, our explanations of the cause of this condition, while expressed differently, are similar. The remedies also set about to achieve the same results through different approaches.

ALOPECIA AREATA, 斑秃 (bān tū) or 鬼剃头 (guǐ tì tóu—literally "ghost-shaved hair") or 光滑头皮风 (guāng huá tóu pí fēng—literally "glossy scalp Wind")
Alopecia areata can occur at any age but is far more common and serious among adults. It does occur sometimes in babies as a small bald spot at the back of the head. This can be aggravated by a calcium deficiency in the baby or in the mother's breast milk. It is an autoimmune disorder and can also be triggered by emotional upheaval or endocrine dysfunction.

When Hair Loss Happens in Babies
对话 (duì huà)
Xiaolan: TCM avoids ingested treatments for babies. I prefer to

recommend massage to increase absorption of vitamins and minerals. Massage has the added bonus of being very pleasurable and increasing the bond between baby and parent. We also seek to correct the breastfeeding mother's diet to ensure that the baby is getting enough calcium. For example, we recommend that she eat Bone Soup (see the recipe on page 99).

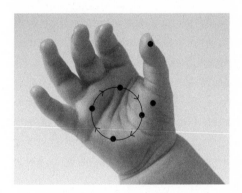

Sandy: In Western medicine, alopecia areata is considered to be an autoimmune disorder in which the body attacks its own hair follicles. I don't worry too much about hair loss in babies under a year old, unless I think it's a symptom of a more generalized and more serious condition that involves the skin, nails and teeth. Later on in childhood, though, alopecia areata can become more than a cosmetic issue if the child is suffering from teasing or other problems. I generally use a topical or injected treatment to counteract the inflammation caused by the autoimmune condition.

Adult Alopecia

In adulthood, alopecia is more widespread and more serious than in children or youngsters. It is often associated with emotional factors and endocrine dysfunction. Whereas in young children it occurs most often in small patches, in adulthood it can result in the loss of all scalp hair, and in cases of alopecia totalis or alopecia universalis, all body hair, including eyebrows, moustache, beard and armpit and pubic hair. Another form of alopecia that is unrelated to autoimmune disease is traumatic alopecia. It can also be caused by habitual hair-pulling, such as from tight hair rollers or constantly wearing the hair in a tight bun or ponytail.

TCM Treatment

It is important not to get the following preparations for hair loss treatment into the eyes. If this happens, immediately rinse them with generous amounts of cold water.

Soothing Scalp Wash

Use this wash once a day for ten days. Do not use shampoo during this time.

25 g	fleeceflower root (*Rx. Polygoni multiflori*, 何首乌, hé shǒu wū)
15 g	red peony root (*Rx. Paeonia rubra*, 赤芍, chì sháo)
15 g	Chinese foxglove, raw (*Rx. Rehmanniae cruda*, 生地黄, shēng dì huáng)
15 g	mulberry mistletoe stems or loranthus (*Viscum coloratum or Taxillus chinensis*, 桑寄生, sāng jì shēng)
10 g	safflower flower, or carthamus (*Fl. Carthemi*, 红花, hóng huā)
10 g	*Saposhnikovia divaricata* root (*Rx. Ledebouriella*, 防风, fáng fēng)
10 g	eclipta (*Hb. Eclipta*, 旱莲草, hàn lián cǎo)
10 g	wild chrysanthemum (*Fl. Chrysanthemi indici*, 野菊花, yě jú huā)
1.5 L	water

In a ceramic, enamel or glass saucepan, combine all the ingredients. Soak for two hours, then bring to a boil and simmer for 45 minutes. Pour through a sieve, reserving the liquid. Discard pulp. Apply the reserved liquid to the hair. Wrap the head in a towel and leave the solution on the hair for one hour. Rinse the hair with clear water.

Golden Shampoo Booster
Make this powder to add to your usual shampoo.

- 50 g   raw Chinese foxglove powder (*Rx. Rehmanniae recens*, 生地黄粉, shēng dì huáng fěn)
- 50 g   sophora root powder (*Rx. Sophora*, 苦参粉, kǔ shēn fěn)
- 20 g   sulphur powder (硫黄粉, liú huáng fěn)

Combine all the ingredients. Store the powder in a sealed jar, and add 2 mL to your shampoo each time you wash your hair.

Root and Flower Tincture for Hair Loss
Apply this tincture morning and night to the affected areas.

- 20 g   ginseng (*Panax ginseng*, 人参, rén shēn)
- 20 g   angelica root (*Rx. Angelica sinensis*, 当归, dāng guī)
- 20 g   Chinese dodder seeds or cuscuta (*Se. Cuscutae*, 菟丝子, tù sī zǐ)
- 20 g   notoginseng (*Panax notoginseng*, 三七, sān qī)
- 15 g   salvia root (*Rx. Salvia*, 丹参, dān shēn)
- 15 g   red peony root (*Rx. Paeonia rubra*, 赤芍, chì sháo)
- 15 g   acanthopanax root bark (*Acanthopanax gracilistylus*, 五加皮, wǔ jiā pí)
- 15 g   notopterygium root (*Rx. Notopterygium incisum*, 羌活, qiāng huó)
- 10 g   safflower flower, or carthamus (*Fl. Carthemi*, 红花, hóng huā)
- 10 g   Szechuan pepper, or zanthoxylum (*Fr. Zanthoxylii*, 川椒, chuān jiāo)
- 500 mL   75 per cent alcohol

Combine all the ingredients and let soak for two weeks before using. The tincture will keep indefinitely at room temperature.

Stinking Rose Rub
Apply this rub to the scalp twice a day.

1   head red garlic (*Allium sativum rubra*, 红皮大蒜, hóng pí dà suàn)

Glycerine (*Symphytum officinalis*, 甘油, gān yóu)

Peel garlic and place in a bowl. With a hand blender, mash it all up. Put the mashed garlic in a piece of cheesecloth and squeeze out the garlic juice into the bowl. Combine the garlic juice with the glycerine in a 3:2 ratio.

Black Silk Chrysalis Tea
Drink 250 mL of this tea in the morning and 250 mL in the evening.

30 g   Chinese foxglove root cooked in wine (*Rx. Rehmanniae conquitae*, 熟地黄, shú dì huáng)

30 g   fleeceflower root (*Rx. Polygoni multiflori*, 何首乌, hé shǒu wū)

30 g   black sesame seeds (*Sesamum indicum nigra*, 黑芝麻, hēi zhī ma)

15 g   angelica root (*Rx. Angelica sinensis*, 当归, dāng guī)

15 g   privet fruit, or ligustrum (*Fr. Ligustri lucidi*, 女贞子, nǚ zhēn zǐ)

15 g   schisandra fruit (*Fr. Schisandra chinensis*, 五味子, wǔ wèi zǐ)

15 g   Chinese yam (*Rx. Dioscorea*, 山药, shān yào)

15 g   white peony root (*Rx. Paeonia alba*, 白芍, bái sháo)

2 L   water

In a ceramic, enamel or glass saucepan, combine all the ingredients.

Let soak for 2 hours, then bring to a boil and simmer for 45 minutes, or until reduced to 500 mL.

对话 (duì huà)

Xiaolan: TCM and Western medicine have quite different views about why hair loss occurs, but this is not necessarily a bad thing—on the contrary. TCM treats hair loss systemically, seeking to cool the Blood and extinguish Wind, nourish Yin and protect the hair. Western medicine treats it locally, with various treatments. Because of these different approaches, hair loss is an instance where TCM and Western treatments can be complementary.

Sandy: In older children or adults with more extensive hair loss, we may try a therapy that confuses the cells in the skin and distracts the immune system from attacking the hair follicle, to give it a chance to recover. In extreme cases such as alopecia totalis or alopecia universalis, we may temporarily suppress the immune system through an oral medication.

My major issue, especially when I see women with hair loss, is to be precise about the type of hair loss that they are experiencing. It's a very emotional subject, so I feel that one of the most important things I do is educate the patient about the reason for their condition. Is it stress? Is it thyroid issues? The reason will determine the treatment. I know we agree that scalp hygiene is important.

Xiaolan: In many patients, hair loss is linked to the thyroid and weight gain. But one of the problems is that lab tests for thyroid issues are so broad. The so-called "normal range" is huge, and sensitivity is highly individual. Supporting Kidney Jing and supplementing iron and iodine are some useful treatments for hair shedding and loss. We agree that it is more important to understand the individual patient than to rely on lab results in these cases.

ANDROGENETIC HAIR LOSS (Thinning), 雄激素性脱发 (xióng jī sù xìng tuō fà)

The gradual hair loss associated with advancing age is quite different from the alopecia problems described above. In TCM, it is the manifestation of the gradual loss of Kidney Qi that comes with the sunset years of the life cycle. TCM will seek to rebuild Kidney Qi to stop the hair loss and to strengthen the remaining hair. If the treatment is undertaken early enough, it can prevent this hair loss altogether.

TCM Treatment

Red Scalp Vigour Tincture

Use this tincture every night to massage the head vigorously until the scalp is red. There is no need to filter the tincture, and it will keep indefinitely at room temperature.

20 g   astragalus (*Rx. Astragali,* 黄芪, huáng qí)

15 g   salvia root (*Rx. Salvia,* 丹参, dān shēn)

15 g   root bark of shaggy-fruited dittany (*Cs. Dictamni,* 白鲜皮, bái xiān pí—literally "white fresh bark")

15 g   vaccaria, or cow cockle (*Se. Vaccariaie,* 王不留行, wáng bù liú xíng)

15 g   eclipta (*Hb. Eclipta,* 旱莲草, hàn lián cǎo)

10 g   Chinese arborvitae twig and leaf (*Cacumen Biotae orientalis ,* 侧柏叶, cè bó yè)

500 mL   95 per cent alcohol

Combine all the ingredients and let soak for two weeks before using.

Daily Black Silk Nourishment Treatment

Drink 250 mL of this in the morning and 250 mL in the evening.

20 g   fleeceflower root (*Rx. Polygoni multiflori,* 何首乌, hé shǒu wū)

15 g   chaenomeles (*Fr. Chaenomeles,* 木瓜, mù guā)

15 g   tall gastrodia tuber (*Rz. Gastrodiae*, 天麻, tiān má)

15 g   Chinese dodder seeds, or cuscuta (*Se. Cuscutae*, 菟丝子, tù sī zǐ)

15 g   albizia bark (*Cortex Albizziae*, 合欢皮, hé huān pí)

15 g   schisandra fruit (*Fr. Schisandra chinensis*, 五味子, wǔ wèi zǐ)

12 g   angelica root (*Rx. Angelica sinensis*, 当归, dāng guī)

12 g   eclipta (*Hb. Eclipta*, 旱莲草, hàn lián cǎo)

12 g   Szechuan lovage root (*Rz. Ligustici Wall.*, 川芎, chuān xiōng)

12 g   *Saposhnikovia divaricata* root (*Rx. Ledebouriella*, 防风, fáng fēng)

12 g   spiny date seed (*Se. Ziziphi spinosae*, 酸枣仁, suān zǎo rén)

2 L   water

In a ceramic, enamel or glass saucepan, combine all the ingredients. Let soak for 2 hours, then bring to a boil and simmer for 45 minutes, or until reduced to 500 mL.

对话 (duì huà)

Sandy: If we could collaborate on this condition, it would be great. So many patients need help with hair loss. My treatment reduces testosterone and increases circulation to the scalp. What does your treatment do?

Xiaolan: When you are dealing with hair, it is always connected to the Kidney. Balance the Kidney, fix the hair.

Sandy: But help me understand this: two people living in the same town, similar in many ways—why does one have hair loss and not the other?

Xiaolan: The truth is, you do see this condition in families. TCM cannot treat genes, but in the argument between nature and nurture, TCM can do a great deal. A good diet and lifestyle and supporting the body's balance and functions can reverse hair loss and many other conditions.

What You Can Do for Androgenetic Hair Loss
Avoid spicy, rich, greasy and sweet foods, and do not drink alcohol.

HANGNAILS (Pyogenic Paronychia)
We often see patients with an inflammation of the skin around the edge of a fingernail or toenail, because a break in the skin has allowed bacteria or yeast to enter and cause infection. Left alone, this condition can result in abscesses, pain, swelling and loss of the nail.

TCM Treatment
Red Dragon Detoxifying Oil
To clear the Heat that is producing the Toxins, clean the area with 75 per cent alcohol, then use this oil to massage the affected area.

30 g	sargentodoxa vine (*Sargentodoxa cuneata*, 红藤, hóng téng)
20 g	ground beetle (*Eupolyphaga*, 土鳖虫, tǔ biēchóng)
20 g	astragalus (*Rx. Astragali*, 黄芪, huáng qí)
20 g	garden burnet root (*Rx. Sanguisorbia*, 地榆, dì yú)
20 g	Chinese rhubarb (*Rx. et Rz. Rhei*, 大黄, dà huáng)
15 g	Szechuan lovage root (*Rz. Ligustici Wall.*, 川芎, chuān xiōng)
15 g	angelica root (*Rx. Angelica sinensis*, 当归, dāng guī)
10 g	dragon blood (*Sanguis draconis*, 血竭, xuè jié)
300 mL	sesame oil (*Sesamum*, 麻油, má yóu)

In a ceramic, enamel or glass saucepan, combine all the ingredients. Cook over low heat until the herbs turn yellow. Pour the oil through a sieve, reserving the oil. Discard the herbs.

对话 (duì huà)

Sandy: Paronychia can be caused by either bacteria or yeast, and these require different treatments. Bacteria can cause an acute infection at the site, and antibiotics such as bacitracin can work. However, if people expose their hangnails to too much moisture, this can trigger a yeast infection. In these cases, we use a topical antifungal such as ciclopirox. If the problem is extreme, we use an oral antifungal.

What You Can Do For Hangnails

Compresses are helpful to draw the infection out of bacterial parony-chias. Avoid too much moisture, as it can lead to yeast infections.

HEAVENLY WATER

In China, everyone in the family understands the importance of taking special care of girls and women during their Heavenly Water. Because prevention and treatment through food are woven into every family's daily life, it is common for Chinese men to have a good understanding of the foods that offer therapeutic value for women's health, and health in general. My father would often make me Egg Soup (see recipe below) from my mother's recipe if he knew that I was menstruating. The soup helps to increase circulation, nourish the body and keep it warm, thus helping the smooth and free movement of Blood and Qi and the harmonious working of the Zang-Fu Organs.

My mother also cooked Sweet Rice Congee (see recipe below), a kind of thin Chinese porridge with dried longan fruit, peanuts and red Chinese dates. The sweet rice helps the energy of the Liver to flow, the longan fruit activates the flow of Qi and increases Blood, and the dates nourish Blood and invigorate the Spleen. Peanuts also benefit the Spleen.

TCM Treatment

Egg Soup

250 mL	water
15 mL	raw cane sugar
2	eggs
45 mL	rice wine

In a medium saucepan, combine the water and raw cane sugar. Bring to a boil over medium-high heat. Crack the eggs into the boiling water and bring back to a boil before adding the rice wine and turning off the heat. Serve warm.
Makes 1 serving.

Sweet Rice Congee

1.5 L	water
250 mL	black sweet rice
125 mL	dried longan fruit (available in Chinese grocery stores)
10	red Chinese dates
25 mL	raw cane sugar
1.5 cm	piece fresh ginger, peeled and thinly sliced

In a large, heavy saucepan, combine the water, black sweet rice, longan fruit, dates and raw cane sugar. Bring to a boil over medium-high heat. Reduce the heat and simmer for 2 hours, stirring occasionally. The finished congee will have the consistency of soup. Ladle it into a bowl and sprinkle with ginger slices.
Makes 4 servings.

HERPES SIMPLEX, 单纯疱疹 (dān chún pào zhěn) or 热疮 (rè chuāng—literally "Heat sore") or 气热疮 (qì rè chuāng—literally "Heat Qi sore")

All forms of herpes simplex are caused by a virus—a simple microscopic invader that attaches itself to healthy cells in the body and takes them over, for its own growth at the expense of its host. There are two widespread forms of herpes simplex: HSV-1, which usually causes oral infections, and HSV-2, associated with genital infections. The virus is highly contagious and usually infects the host in two phases, often beginning in childhood.

The first round of infection can be deceptive, because it causes skin infections that heal without scarring, usually around the mouth. The virus remains lurking in the system, however, waiting for a chance to return. Once it is reactivated, sometimes by trauma (a cut, exposure to radiation or too much sun) or systemic problems (febrile illness, respiratory infection, fatigue or stress, or menstruation), the virus travels along the nerves to cause a secondary infection at the original site. This kind of infection can strike any skin surface or mucous membrane in the body. The lesions of the primary infection usually last about two weeks but can take six weeks to heal. The recurrent sores that come with the secondary infection are neither as serious nor as long-lasting as the primary ones, but they can itch, burn or tingle. In TCM, the primary cause of herpes simplex is exuberant Heat with Wind Qi (pathogenic Wind).

In TCM, herpes eruptions constitute an Excess-Heat pattern. The short-lived skin lesions can be severe, burning and tingling, with occasional fever and coughing. The treatment seeks to dissipate Wind and clear Heat, transform Dampness and relieve Toxicity. Sometimes the disease can be persistent. In this case, TCM explains it through a Qi and Yin Deficiency. In these cases, we seek to augment the Qi and nourish Yin, support Vital Qi (Zheng Qi) and consolidate the Root. This condition requires patience, as the treatment can take two months.

TCM Treatment

Treasure Herb and Root Wash

Wash the affected areas directly with this solution two or three times a day. It does not need refrigeration.

- 20 g   pomegranate husk (*Punica granatum,* 石榴皮, shí liú pí)
- 20 g   garden burnet root (*Rx. Sanguisorbia,* 地榆, dì yú)
- 20 g   cnidium (*Se. Cnidium,* 蛇床子, shé chuáng zǐ)
- 20 g   dandelion (*Hb. Tara,* 蒲公英, pú gōng yīng)
- 20 g   sophora root (*Rx. Sophora,* 苦参, kǔ shēn)
- 2 L   water

In a ceramic, enamel or glass saucepan, combine all the ingredients. Let soak for 2 hours, then bring to a boil and simmer for 40 minutes.

Heavenly Calming Powder

Apply this powder to the affected areas as needed.

- 20 g   amur cork tree bark powder (*Cx. Phellodendri,* 黄柏粉, huáng bǎi fěn)
- 10 g   Chinese wild ginger powder (*Asarum sieboldii,* 细辛粉, xì xīn fěn)
- 10 g   realgar powder (*Realgar,* 雄黄粉, xióng huáng fěn)
- 5 g   calomel powder (*Calomelas,* 轻 粉, qīng fěn)

Combine all the ingredients. Store the powder in a sealed jar at room temperature.

Calming Green Goddess Herbal Bath for Herpes

- 50 g   lotus leaf (*Nelumbo nucifera,* 荷叶, hé yè)
- 30 g   green tea (*Camellia sinensis,* 绿茶, lǜ chá)
- 2   bunches fresh coriander (*Coriandrum sativum,* 香菜, xiāng cài)

Add all the ingredients to very hot bathwater. When the bath has cooled enough, sit in it for 20 minutes.

Night and Day Healing Paste for Herpes
Apply this paste to the lesions as needed.

- 20 g   realgar powder (*Realgar*, 雄黄粉, xióng huáng fěn)
- 20 g   indigo root powder (*Rx. Indigo naturalis*, 青黛 粉, qīng dài fěn)
- 2 g   borneol powder (*Dryobalanops aromatica* or *Blumea balsamifera*, 冰片粉, bīng piàn fěn)
-         Rice vinegar

Combine all the powders with enough rice vinegar to make a paste. Store in a sealed jar at room temperature.

Parents should use only the following massage treatments on babies and young children.

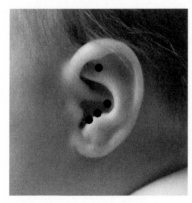 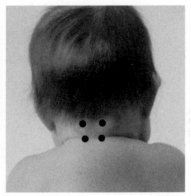

对话 (duì huà)

Sandy: Xiaolan, in the area of primary treatment, I am struck by the commonalities between Western medicine and TCM. For example, we would both agree that wet compresses are recommended to soothe the skin lesions when they are inflamed.

Although herpes does not require treatment, it does remain dormant in the nerve ganglion once you have had it. For the general population, this is not overly serious. However, for those whose immune systems are compromised, such as HIV-positive or cancer patients, we treat this viral infection with anti-herpes medications, either topically or orally—and we sometimes save their lives. You may know these under brand names such as Zovirax, Valtrex and Famvir.

Xiaolan: This is a case where Western medicine will help with the active phases of the disease, while TCM will help prevent recurrences.

What You Can Do for Herpes Simplex

When the viral infection is active, avoid skin-to-skin contact with others. Avoid stress, get lots of rest and eat properly to avoid recurrence of the sores. Wet compresses can help to soothe the lesions.

HERPES ZOSTER

See Shingles on page 170.

INTERTRIGO, 间擦疹 (jiān cā zhěn) or 汗水浸泡疮 (hàn shuǐ jìn pào chuāng—literally "sweat immersion sore")

Intertrigo is a redness and irritation of skin folds, sometimes weepy and shiny, in areas such as underarms and under the breasts, and can spread. In babies, it can be mistaken for common diaper rash. It is caused by friction or sweating, and can be complicated by candida infection.

Intertrigo can happen at any age if people have folds in their skin due to obesity, if they wear overly tight clothing, exercise poor personal hygiene, have diabetes mellitus or suffer from general weakness due to illness. If it is complicated by *Candida albicans*, intertrigo can even show up in the webs between the fingers of people whose hands are often in water. The condition starts with a slight inflammation or swelling and develops into pustules and red glazed plaques. There may be moist scaling at the margins of the plaques. As the condition progresses, the sores get worse and more painful. They cause a burning sensation, itching and a stabbing pain where the skin erodes.

TCM Treatment

The principle of the treatment is to clear Heat and cool the Blood, transforming the Dampness and relieving Toxicity and pain. With babies, it is very important to bring the condition under control as soon as possible. It is difficult to get babies to ingest herbs, although a breastfeeding mother may take them to influence the baby's condition. See the treatment for diaper rash, starting on page 112.

M

MEASLES, 麻疹 (má zhěn)

Measles provides a striking example of the difference between TCM and Western treatment approaches. Measles is an acute infectious disease—serious and potentially fatal in many poor countries—but it has become much less common in Western countries because of mass immunization. However, now that the rates of immunization are falling, it is possible that we will see a resurgence of measles.

Measles is caused by the RNA virus passing through the respiratory tract and by seasonal epidemic Toxins, and is Yang in nature. It occurs mostly in children between six months and five years of age. Newborn babies acquire passive immunity from their mothers (if they have it) for the first three or four months of life, but it wears off over time. Symptoms appear nine to eleven days after exposure, on average, and the disease lasts about two weeks. Measles is more likely to spread in winter and spring.

Young children have weak defence systems against Yang disease because the Qi of their Zang-Fu Organs is not strong and their bodies are full of Yang Qi, which combines with the Yang disease to affect the body. This causes Heat to ferment and transform into Fire, which leads to a range of Warm-Febrile symptoms. During the phase when the spots are erupting, there may be a high fever—sometimes, alarmingly, as high as forty-one degrees Celsius—watery eyes and light sensitivity, a runny nose with sticky discharge, coughing, and sometimes digestive problems such as nausea, vomiting and diarrhea. Small red spots with white centres may appear inside the mouth first, before a rosy rash erupts along the hairline and on the face and spreads rapidly to the neck, upper limbs, trunk and lower limbs.

(If you press these spots, they briefly turn white.) Such high fevers often come with enlarged lymph nodes in the neck, liver and spleen.

Once the fever begins to subside (beginning about a week after it appears or slightly sooner), the rash gradually turns dark brown, then scaly, before disappearing. Complications following measles can be serious, including tidal fever, diarrhea or dysentery, and suppurative inflammation of the cheek and mouth.

TCM Treatment

Royal Bath for Measles

Bathe with this solution once a day for 5 days.

- 50 g   water chestnuts (*Eleocharis dulcis*, 马蹄, mǎ tí)
- 50 g   red carrots (*Daucus carota* var. *sativa*, 红胡萝卜, hóng hú luó bo)
- 30 g   goldenseal, or Chinese goldthread root (*Rz. Coptidis*, 黄连根, huáng lián gēn)
- 30 g   belvedere fruit (*Fr. Kochia*, 地肤子, dì fū zǐ)
- 2 L   water
- 10 g   alum (*Potassium Aluminum Sulphate*, 明矾, míng fán)

In a ceramic, enamel or glass saucepan, combine the water chestnuts, carrots, goldenseal, belvedere fruit and water. Let soak for 2 hours, then bring to a boil and simmer for 30 minutes. Pour it through a sieve, reserving the liquid. Add the alum to the reserved liquid, and then add the alum mixture to the bathwater.

Fresh Wind Tincture

Apply this tincture to the lesions three times a day. It is also useful for insect bites (from mosquitoes, bed bugs, fleas, etc.).

- 20 g   camphor (*Cx. Cinnamomi camphora*, 樟脑, zhāng nǎo)
- 20 g   menthol (*Mentha arvensis*, 薄荷, bò hé)
- 20 g   amur cork tree bark powder (*Cx. Phellodendri*, 黄柏粉, huáng bǎi fěn)

20 g   Baikal skullcap (*Rx. Scutellariae*, 黄芩, huáng qín)

15 g   senecio, or climbing groundsel (*Senecio cineraria*, 千里光, qiān lǐ guāng)

200 mL   75 per cent alcohol

Soak the herbs in the alcohol for 2 days before using. The tincture need not be filtered and will keep indefinitely at room temperature.

Parents can also massage the child.

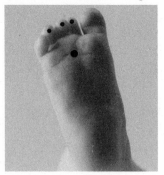 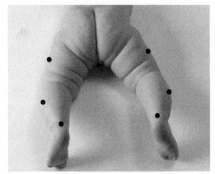

对话 (duì huà)

Sandy: Measles has become so rare in the West that I have never had to treat it. I do tell parents that it is important to determine whether a child has measles, roseola, rubella (which is dangerous to pregnant women) or some other viral disease. Since the complications of measles include ear infections, pneumonia and encephalitis in one in a thousand cases, and potentially death in HIV-infected children, the price of refusing immunization seems excessively high. The Western approach is to treat the symptoms: control the fever, rinse the mouth for the spots, and use antibiotics if there is a secondary infection.

Xiaolan: I am concerned about the non-medicinal ingredients in vaccines. A balanced body is able to fight the disease without this assistance.

Sandy: I disagree. The ratio of complications from the vaccine is ten to eighteen times lower than for the disease.

Xiaolan: Having looked at the statistics, I am prepared to say that although I still have reservations about many vaccines, I recognize that the potential for neurological damage is too high to risk in the case of measles.

Sandy: Some North American parents who have your concerns ask to have their babies vaccinated for measles, but not for mumps and rubella. The vaccines usually come packaged as a single inoculation known as MMR.

What You Can Do for Measles
With measles patients, the skin should be kept clean and dry. If the eyes are sensitive, keep the child in a darkened room. Lots of water, soups and light meals are best.

MELANOMA
See Skin Cancer, page 171.

MELASMA, or CHLOASMA, 黄褐斑 (huáng hè bān or mian chen—literally "dusty complexion")
There are many factors that determine the pigmentation in the skin and subcutaneous tissues. The melanocytes in the basal layer of the epidermis produce melanin that determines skin colour; carotene in the stratum corneum and subcutaneous fat, along with oxyhemoglobin in the blood, also change skin tones. Where the skin is thick, it appears darker and lacks transparency; where it is thin, it takes on the colour of the blood in the small vessels beneath. Other factors such as drug use, tattoos, metals, cosmetics, metabolic pigments

from diseases such as jaundice, and changes related to illness such as thickening, swelling, inflammation or dead tissue can all affect the skin pigmentation.

Hyperactivity of the melanocytes can lead to melasma (also known as chloasma) due to changes in the endocrine gland system. Underactivity of the melanocytes can happen in atopic eczema, pityriasis alba, psoriasis and post-inflammatory hypopigmentation. In some diseases, such as vitiligo and halo nevus, there can be a depigmentation caused by a loss of melanocyte cells. Albinism, a condition in which the skin makes little or no melanin, can be triggered by an abnormality in the body's management of an amino acid called tyrosine.

Many pregnant women experience what is known as the "mask of pregnancy"—a discoloration of the skin causing yellow or brown patches on the face. It is the result of a combination of estrogen levels, sun exposure and nervous disorders. Melasma tends to affect pregnant women in the second and third trimesters, women taking oral contraceptives, and people with darker skin. Pigmentation is symmetrical, mainly on the forehead and cheeks, around the mouth and nose, and on the chin. The lesions can become darker and larger during pregnancy but turn lighter or disappear after birth, after stopping contraceptives, or in the recovery phase of liver disease. The pigment changes happen slowly and are more obvious after exposure to sunlight.

TCM Treatment

TCM attributes these spots to Blood and Qi deficiency, as well as a Kidney Yin deficiency, a result of nourishing the baby during pregnancy. The spots can be stress-related. While they are most common in pregnant women, they can also occur in older people, unrelated to pregnancy.

Pure White Gel Face Mask

Use this mask daily as long as the problem persists. It is also excellent for liver spots and other pigment disorders.

    20 g   white peony root powder (*Rx. Paeonia alba*, 白芍粉, bái sháo fěn)

    20 g   dahurian angelica powder (*Rx. Angelica dahurica*, 白芷粉, bái zhǐ fěn)

    20 g   white chrysanthemum powder (*Fl. Chrysanthemi alba*, 白菊花粉, bái jú huā fěn)

    20 g   stiff silkworm powder (*Bombyx batryticatus*, 僵蚕粉, jiāng cán fěn)

    20 g   salvia root powder (*Rx. Salvia*, 丹参粉, dān shēn fěn)

    20 g   skin of the tree peony root, or moutan powder (*Cx. Moutan radicis rubra*, 牡丹皮粉, mǔ dān pí fěn)

    1   egg white

Combine all the ingredients and apply to affected areas. Leave on for 15 minutes, then rinse gently with clear, lukewarm water.

Healing Root Massage Oil

    20 g   giant typhonium rhizome powder (*Rz. Typhonii*, 白附子粉, bái fù zǐ fěn)

    15 g   Thunberg fritillary bulb (*Bo. Fritillariae Thunbergii*, 浙贝母粉, zhè bèi mǔ fěn)

    5 g   sulphur powder (硫黄粉, liú huáng fěn)

    2 g   borneol powder (*Dryobalanops aromatica* or *Blumea balsamifera*, 冰片粉, bīng piàn fěn)

    200 mL   sesame oil (*Sesamum*, 麻油, má yóu)

Combine all the ingredients and let soak for 1 week. Warm the oil before using it to massage the face and any other affected areas as needed.

Smoothing Pigment Herbal Tea

Drink 250 mL of this tea in the morning and 250 mL in the evening.

15 g	Chinese foxglove, raw (*Rx. Rehmanniae recens,* 生地黄, shēng dì huáng)
15 g	angelica root (*Rx. Angelica sinensis,* 当归, dāng guī)
15 g	bupleurum (*Rx. Bupleuri,* 柴胡, chái hú)
15 g	poria (*Poria,* 茯苓, fú ling)
15 g	gromwell root (*Rx. Lithospermum,* 紫草根, zǐ cǎo gēn)
15 g	Chinese yam (*Rx. Dioscorea,* 山药, shān yào)
12 g	cornelian cherry (*Fr. Corni officinalis,* 山茱萸, shān zhū yú)
10 g	red peony root (*Rx. Paeonia rubra,* 赤芍, chì sháo)
10 g	Szechuan lovage root (*Rz. Ligustici Wall.,* 川芎, chuān xiōng)
10 g	peach kernel (*Se. Persica,* 桃仁, táo rén)
10 g	safflower flower, or carthamus (*Fl. Carthemi,* 红花, hóng huā)
10 g	alisma (*Rz. Alismatic,* 泽泻, zé xiè)
2 L	water

In a ceramic, enamel or glass saucepan, combine all the ingredients. Let soak for 2 hours, then bring to a boil and simmer for 45 minutes, or until reduced to 500 mL.

对话 (duì huà)

Sandy: Western medicine views melasma as one of the more stubborn problems to remedy. We use a combination of sunscreen and various treatments. The condition takes time to treat and may recur. We use hydroquinone, a medication that inhibits tyrosinase, an enzyme that is necessary for the production of melanin. We also use creams based on glycolic or retinoic acid. Azelaic acid is a new formulation that shows promise in decreasing melanin synthesis. Kojic acid and ascorbic acid (vitamin C) may also offer some assistance with melasma.

Chemical peels with lactic acid, glycolic acid or trichloroacetic acid may help to mitigate the condition. Intense pulsed light (IPL) or fractional lasers are the other options when all else fails. Fractional lasers can be very effective with this condition.

Xiaolan: I do not see the need for such harsh intervention. I believe that gentler preparations and TCM approaches can help balance the body to attenuate this purely cosmetic condition.

What You Can Do for Melasma
It is important to use an SPF 60 sunscreen with a broad range of UVA and UVB filtration ability, every day, rain or shine. If the condition is bad and you are taking an oral contraceptive, you may need to stop taking it to see an improvement.

MENSTRUAL CRAMPS
See Heavenly Water, page 135.

MOLES
See Skin Cancer, page 171.

MORNING SICKNESS
During pregnancy, women often experience morning sickness or nausea. This is generally an expression of blocked Stomach Qi. Ginger is one of the best remedies for this, and can restore a woman's balance and comfort when she is Ripening the Fruit.

TCM Treatment
Ginger and Mint Tea
  2.5 cm   piece fresh ginger root, peeled and grated
  5 leaves   fresh mint

    1 L   boiling water
          Honey

Place the ginger and mint in a teapot. Pour boiling water over, cover and steep for 3 to 5 minutes before serving. Add honey to taste.
Makes 8 servings.

Ginger and Orange Tea
  1.5 cm   piece fresh ginger root, peeled and grated
    7 mL   grated orange rind
      1 L   boiling water
          Honey

Place the ginger and grated orange peel in a teapot. Pour boiling water over, cover and allow to steep for 3 to 5 minutes before serving. Add honey to taste.
Makes 8 servings.

Ginger Rice
     1   large, fresh ginger root
  250 mL   cooked rice

Peel the ginger root and cut it up into rough chunks. Place the ginger in a bowl and, with a hand blender, mash it up. Put the mashed ginger in a piece of cheesecloth and squeeze out the ginger juice into the bowl. You should have 5 mL of ginger juice. Put the rice in a medium skillet over low heat. Sprinkle the ginger juice over the rice and stir-fry it until the rice turns yellow, about 5 minutes. Chewing the rice will help alleviate nausea.
Makes 1 serving.

N

NAIL INFECTIONS

Another source of fungal and yeast infections is the practice of covering natural nails with false ones that do not breathe, for years on end. Over time, the nail bed becomes soft and vulnerable to these invasions. Teenaged girls are especially vulnerable to nail infections, as many cover their nails with acrylic or other materials that stop the tissues from breathing.

TCM Treatment

Return to Health Manicure Wash

Soak the nails in this wash twice a day.

20 g	sophora root (*Rx. Sophora*, 苦参, kǔ shēn)
15 g	amur cork tree bark (*Cx. Phellodendri*, 黄柏, huáng bǎi)
15 g	chaulmoogra seeds, or hydnocarpus (*Se. Hydnocarpus*, 大枫子, dà fēng zǐ)
10 g	realgar (*Realgar*, 雄黄, xióng huáng)
10 g	Szechuan pepper, or zanthoxylum (*Fr. Zanthoxylii*, 川椒, chuān jiāo)
10 g	alum (*Potassium Aluminum Sulphate*, 明矾, míng fán)
6 g	licorice (*Rx. Glycyrrhizae*, 甘草, gān cǎo)
2 L	water
	Rice vinegar

In a ceramic, enamel or glass saucepan, combine all the herbs with the water. Soak for 2 hours, then bring to a boil and simmer for 45 minutes. Pour through a sieve, reserving the liquid. Discard the pulp. Measure the amount of liquid and add the same amount of rice vinegar. This wash can be stored at room temperature and reused for three days before discarding it.

Spicy Tincture for Nails
Apply this tincture to the nail beds twice a day.

20 g Szechuan pepper, or zanthoxylum (*Fr. Zanthoxylii*, 川椒, chuān jiāo)

20 g hydnocarpus (*Se. Hydnocarpus*, 大枫子, dà fēng zǐ)

10 g realgar powder (*Realgar*, 雄黄粉, xióng huáng fěn)

10 g pseudolaric hibiscus bark (*Cx. Pseudolaricis*, 土荆皮, tǔ jīng pí)

200 mL 75 per cent alcohol

Combine all the ingredients and let soak for 1 week before using. The tincture can keep at room temperature indefinitely.

对话 (duì huà)

Sandy: I discourage all my patients from wearing false nails—not only because of the danger from potential fungus or yeast infections, but also because the acrylate in the false nails triggers allergic contact dermatitis in some patients. Developing an allergy to acrylate is a bad idea, because later in life, you might need this substance for use in bonding teeth.

If patients do get a nail infection, it is important to do a culture to identify the cause, because the treatment—usually an oral antifungal—is specific to each yeast or fungus. I have had some success with a topical antifungal nail lacquer.

P

PHOTO DAMAGE
See under Sunburn, page 187.

PITYRIASIS ALBA, 白色糠疹 (bái sè kāng zhěn) or 褐色花癣 (hé sè huā xiǎn—literally "brown blossom tinea")

This condition often appears in spring on the faces of children and young adults in the form of dry, superficial, flat dark patches that shed dry skin. It is more common in spring, but most visible in summer, when the patches do not tan. The patches appear most frequently around the mouth and on the chin, cheeks and forehead, and less frequently on the neck, shoulder, upper arm or thigh. Lesions are usually white or pale pink, covered with fine, dry scales. If they are very dry, they may be slightly itchy.

TCM Treatment

Brown Blossom Bath

Sponge-bathe with this solution. It is suitable for babies and young children.

50 g	honeysuckle flower (*Fl. Lonicera*, 金银花, jīn yín huā)
30 g	licorice (*Rx. Glycyrrhizae*, 甘草, gān cǎo)
30 g	dandelion (*Hb. Tara*, 蒲公英, pú gōng yīng)
2 L	water

In a ceramic, enamel or glass saucepan, combine all the ingredients. Let soak for 2 hours, then bring to a boil and simmer for 20 minutes.

Brown Blossom Massage Oil

This massage oil is suitable for babies and young children.

20 g	gypsum fibrosum powder (*Gypsum fibrosum*, 石膏粉, shí gāo fěn)
20 g	talcum powder (*Talcum*, 滑石粉, huá shí fěn)
10 g	indigo root powder (*Rx. Indigo naturalis*, 青黛粉, qīng dài fěn)
10 g	amur cork tree bark powder (*Cx. Phellodendri*, 黄柏粉, huáng bǎi fěn)
200 mL	sesame oil (*Sesamum*, 麻油, má yóu)

Combine all the ingredients and let soak for 2 days before using. Massage the child's Meridians following the directions below.

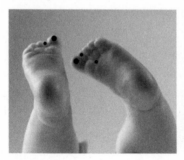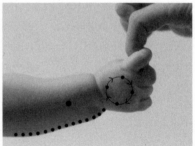

对话 (duì huà)

Sandy: Pityriasis alba is a minor form of atopic dermatitis that results in an irritation of the melanocytes, the cells that produce pigment in the skin. The irritation debilitates the cells, resulting in white patches on the skin. The Latin translation means "white scaly patches." We see it frequently in young children and adolescents, mostly on the face, but sometimes on the arms. Essentially, people outgrow it, and attempts to treat it are often the equivalent of shutting the door after the horse has left the barn. By the time the patches are white, it is too late. I tell people to use corticosteroid cream on the sites as soon as they appear dry and scaly.

Xiaolan: In TCM, we believe that the skin is always expressing something that is going on inside the body. If I see a child developing this condition, I will provide herbs for the parents to treat it.

PSORIASIS, 银屑病 (yín xiè bìng) or 白壳 (bái ké—literally "white crust") or 牛皮癣 (niú pí xiǎn—literally "silver crumbs disease")

Psoriasis is a chronic inflammatory disease in which the skin develops large silvery white scales. Up to 3 per cent of the world's population suffers from the disease, although it is more common in Europe and North America than in Africa and Asia. The reason for the scaly tissue is that the cells in the stratum corneum (the horny outer layer) of the skin begin to multiply more than three times faster than the rest of the skin—over four days instead of the normal fourteen. This results in an excess number of these scaly cells, which appear as psoriatic plaques. There is often a hereditary factor—a person has a 15 to 25 per cent chance of developing the disease if one parent has it, and a 50 to 60 per cent chance if both parents have it. Although psoriasis is not contagious, infection may play a role, as do stress, trauma, environmental factors, and drug reactions.

Psoriasis can start at any age (but rarely under ten years of age), peaking between fifteen and thirty years and again between fifty-five and sixty years. The most common places for the scales are the elbows and knees, the lower back and the scalp. There are several types of psoriasis, including guttate (associated with group A streptococcal infections and most often found in adolescents and young adults); flexural (usually in older people, and more often in women than men); pustular (rare); erythrodermic (a serious disease requiring hospital treatment); and psoriatic arthritis (in up to 5 per cent of cases, which is higher in colder climates).

While psoriasis is normally a disease that ebbs and flows, it can evolve over time into a persistent, ongoing condition. When this happens, the texture of the skin itself changes. The condition drains the patient's energy. It is important to make a special effort to remain fit, avoid upper respiratory infections and increase the intake of fresh fruits and vegetables.

In China, patients with severe psoriasis are sent to an area with hot sulphurous springs, with very beneficial effects. In general, dry heat and vitamin D are helpful to psoriasis patients. Psoriasis can be a difficult disease to endure, and some patients find consolation in alcohol. This can lead to a "chicken and egg" situation in which the alcohol consumption aggravates the psoriasis and the worsening disease drives the patient to drink more. Psoriasis patients may need support to keep this problem under control and to prevent aggravation of their condition.

TCM Treatment for Psoriasis in Adults

Treatment may involve wash preparations, ointments, acupuncture, moxibustion therapy and, in some cases, hospitalization in conjunction with treatment by Western medicine.

Herbal Mineral Wash

Sponge-bathe the affected areas directly with this solution once a day.

30 g	vaccaria, or cow cockle (*Se. Vaccaria*, 王不留行, wáng bù liú xíng)
30 g	Chinese arborvitae twig and leaf (*Cacumen Biotae orientalis*, 侧柏叶, cè bó yè)
25 g	mirabilite, or Glauber's salt (*Mirabilitum*, 芒硝, máng xiāo)
20 g	garden burnet root (*Rx. Sanguisorbia*, 地榆, dì yú)
20 g	catmint (*Hb. Schizonepeta*, 荆芥, jīng jiè)
2 L	water

In a ceramic, enamel or glass saucepan, combine all the ingredients. Let soak for 2 hours, then bring to a boil and simmer for 40 minutes. Store in the refrigerator.

Aromatic Healing Belly-Button Paste

Place a small amount of this paste in or around the navel, changing it twice a day.

15 g belvedere fruit powder (*Fr. Kochia*, 地肤子粉, dì fū zǐ fěn)

15 g trichosanthes root powder (*Rx. Trichosanthis*, 天花粉, tiān huā fěn—literally "heavenly flower powder")

15 g salvia root powder (*Rx. Salvia*, 丹参粉, dān shēn fěn)

2 g borneol powder (*Dryobalanops aromatica or Blumea balsamifera*, 冰片粉, bīng piàn fěn)

Olive oil (*Olea europaea*, 橄榄油, gǎn lǎn yóu)

Combine all the ingredients to make a paste. Store in a sealed jar at room temperature.

Strong Blue Healing Paste

Apply this paste directly to the lesions twice a day.

20 g sulphur powder (硫黄粉, liú huáng fěn)

20 g indigo root powder (*Rx. Indigo naturalis*, 青黛粉, qīng dài fěn)

15 g smithsonite or calamine powder (*Smithsonitum*, 炉甘石粉, lú gān shí fěn)

Sesame oil (*Sesamum*, 麻油, má yóu)

Combine all the powders with enough sesame oil to make a paste.

Robust Healing Tea

Drink 250 mL of this tea in the morning and 250 mL in the evening.

15 g Chinese foxglove, raw (*Rx. Rehmanniae recens*, 生地黄, shēng dì huáng)

15 g	gromwell root (*Rx. Lithospermum*, 紫草, zǐ cǎo)
15 g	salvia root (*Rx. Salvia*, 丹参, dān shēn)
12 g	red peony root (*Rx. Paeonia rubra*, 赤芍, chì sháo)
12 g	ningpo figwort (*Rx. Scrophuloriae*, 玄参, xuán shēn)
12 g	skin of the tree peony root, or moutan (*Cx. Moutan radicis rubra*, 牡丹皮, mǔ dān pí)
10 g	pagoda tree flower (*Rx. Sophora*, 槐花, huái huā)
10 g	Chinese rhubarb (*Rx. et Rz. Rhei*, 大黄, dà huáng)
10 g	safflower flower or carthamus (*Fl. Carthemi*, 红花, hóng huā)
2 L	water

In a ceramic, enamel or glass saucepan, combine all the ingredients. Let soak for 2 hours, then bring to a boil and simmer for 45 minutes, or until reduced to 500 mL.

Pearly Grit Face Mask
If the psoriasis is on the face, prepare this cooling mask and apply it once a day for 20 minutes. Rinse gently with clear, lukewarm water.

25 g	apricot seed powder (*Se. Pruni armeniacae*, 杏仁粉, xìng rén fěn)
25 g	peppermint powder (*Hb. Menthae*, 薄荷 粉, bò he fěn)
25 g	pearl powder (*Con. Margarita*, 珍珠粉, zhēn zhū fěn)
200 mL	glycerine (*Symphytum officinalis*, 甘油, gān yóu)

Combine all the ingredients and apply to the face.

White Veil Bath

25 g	sophora root (*Rx. Sophora*, 苦参, kǔ shēn)
25 g	cnidium (*Se. Cnidium*, 蛇床子, shé chuáng zǐ)
20 g	root bark of shaggy-fruited dittany (*Cs. Dictamni*, 白鲜皮, bái xiān pí—literally "white fresh bark")
10 g	sulphur (硫黄, liú huáng)

10 g   burnt alum powder (*Potassium Aluminum Sulphate* 烧
明矾粉, shāo míng fán fěn)

2 L   water

In a ceramic, enamel or glass saucepan, combine all the ingredients.
Let soak for 2 hours, then bring to a boil and simmer for 45 minutes.
Pour through a sieve, reserving the liquid. Discard the pulp. Use the
liquid to sponge-bathe the affected areas once a day. This preparation does not require refrigeration.

Eastern Promise Cream

Use this cream to massage the affected skin three times a day.
It is most effective used after White Veil Bath, but it may also be
used on its own.

30 g   apricot seed powder (*Se. Pruni armeniacae*, 杏仁粉,
xìng rén fěn)

20 g   sulphur powder (硫黄粉, liú huáng fěn)

20 g   frankincense powder (*Boswellia carterii*, 乳香粉, rǔ
xiāng fěn—literally "fragrant milk")

20 g   myrrh powder (*Commiphora myrrh*, 没药粉, mò yào fěn)

10 g   alum powder (*Potassium Aluminum Sulphate*, 明矾粉,
míng fán fěn)

300 mL   sesame oil (*Sesamum*, 麻油, má yóu)

Combine all the ingredients to make a cream. Store tightly covered
at room temperature.

Silver Hope Tea

Drink 250 mL of this tea in the morning and 250 mL in the evening.

20 g   Chinese foxglove, raw (*Rx. Rehmanniae recens*, 生地
黄, shēng dì huáng)

15 g   Chinese clematis root (*Rx. Clematidis*, 威灵仙, wēi
líng xiān)

15 g suberect spatholobus stem (*Cs. Spatholboli*, 鸡血藤, jī xuè téng)

15 g puncture vine (*Fr. Tribulus terrestris*, 白蒺藜, bái jí lí)

2 L water

In a ceramic, enamel or glass saucepan, combine all the ingredients. Let soak for 2 hours, then bring to a boil and simmer for 45 minutes, or until reduced to 500 mL.

TCM Treatment for Psoriasis in Children

Spice Flower Wash

Sponge-bathe with this solution daily for one week.

30 g cinnamon twig (*Cx. Cinnamomi*, 桂枝, guì zhī)

20 g sophora root (*Rx. Sophora*, 苦参, kǔ shēn)

20 g fleeceflower root (*Rx. Polygori multiflori*, 何首乌, hé shǒu wū)

2 L water

In a ceramic, enamel or glass saucepan, combine all the ingredients. Let soak for 2 hours, then bring to a boil and simmer for 30 minutes.

Silver Scale Tincture

Apply this tincture to the lesions twice a day.

30 g pseudolaric hibiscus bark (*Cx. Pseudolaricis*, 土荆皮, tǔ jīng pí)

20 g Chinese rhubarb (*Rx. et Rz. Rhei*, 大黄, dà huáng)

20 g cnidium (*Se. Cnidium*, 蛇床子, shé chuáng zǐ)

500 mL 75 per cent alcohol

Combine all the ingredients and let soak for 3 days before using. The tincture will keep indefinitely at room temperature.

Dream Oil for Children

Massage the child once a day with this preparation.

25 g	gromwell root (*Rx. Lithospermum*, 紫草根, zǐ cǎo gēn)
25 g	myrrh (*Commiphora myrrha*, 没药, mò yào)
20 g	frankincense (*Boswellia carterii*, 乳香, rǔ xiāng)
20 g	almond (*Amygdalus communis*, 杏仁, xìng rén)
10 g	alum (*Potassium Aluminum Sulphate*, 明矾, míng fán)
300 mL	sesame oil (*Sesamum*, 麻油, má yóu)

Combine all the ingredients and let soak for 7 days. Pour the oil through a sieve to remove the herbs.

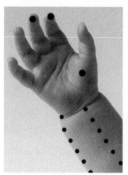 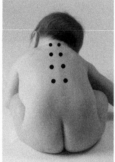 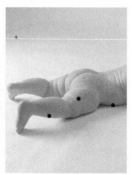

对话 (duì huà)

Sandy: The Western view is that psoriasis is a recurrent chronic scaly condition, although it can lead to the more serious condition of psoriatic arthritis. We have a number of medications and techniques to alleviate the symptoms, but little to cure the underlying condition. I tend to tailor psoriasis treatments to the patient's attitude toward their situation. For example, if it is cosmetically unacceptable and is interfering with the patient's ability to work, socialize or be intimate with a partner, I will design a more aggressive treatment. For example, one of my patients, a senior businessman with significant public speaking and representational responsibilities, had psoriasis of the nails. He was acutely self-conscious about his condition and asked for help. Although this is unusual, I prescribed a course of oral medication that would be considered aggressive for a relatively minor form of psoriasis. One of my patients who has widespread psoriasis is not concerned with the aesthetics, and only wants help with the severe dryness that it provokes. For him, I provide what I consider to be the best medicated lotion, and leave it at that.

Xiaolan: In TCM, psoriasis is considered a systemic disease. In particular, psoriasis treatment for older people will focus more on the problem of Blood Stasis, as the condition has frequently been allowed to go on for too long.

Sandy: Western practitioners do not distinguish psoriasis treatment by age group. However, sometimes older patients develop other illnesses that force us to restrict their access to contraindicated medications that would otherwise be useful to treat psoriasis, and this can be challenging. Conversely, medications that are commonly used among older patients, such as beta blockers and ASA, can worsen the condition.

Some patients find that psoriasis settles down in old age; others find that it becomes increasingly severe and chronic. I have noticed that some of my menopausal patients who are stressed experience flares in their psoriasis at this time in their lives. I think you can help these patients a lot, Xiaolan.

Xiaolan: I see that in my practice too, but I think that it bears out the idea that this is a disease with much deeper and broader causes than the superficial ones. But I also think that in cases where the disease is flaring acutely, your interventions can be very useful. Psoriasis is a disease where Western and TCM therapies are complementary.

What You Can Do for Psoriasis

Avoid respiratory infections, stress, fatigue and excessive consumption of alcohol. Aspirin, beta blockers, lithium and some anti-inflammatories aggravate psoriasis and should be avoided if possible. Increase your intake of fresh fruits and vegetables, and maintain your overall level of fitness.

PYOGENIC PARONYCHIA

See Hangnails, page 134.

R

RADIODERMATITIS, 放射性皮炎 (fàng shè xìng pí yán)

Radiation is often part of the treatment for breast cancer—and many other forms of cancer. When the skin is repeatedly exposed to radiation, inflammation sets in. It is usually classified in three levels: mild, moderate and severe.

In mild radiodermatitis, the skin is bright red initially and then evolves into dull red patches with mild swelling. There may be a sensation of scorching heat and itching. The skin may peel and change colour over three to six weeks.

In moderate radiodermatitis, the lesions are acutely inflamed and swollen. The skin is tense and shiny. Blisters may form, with erosion when they burst. These lesions heal within one to three months, and there will generally be permanent marking, colour changes and visible changes in small blood vessels just beneath the surface.

In severe radiodermatitis, lesions and swelling may be followed by death of the tissues. Persistent ulcerating sores form to different depths of tissue. There will also be headaches, dizziness, listlessness and many other side effects, as well as a decrease in the white blood cell count.

Radiodermatitis may also be chronic, most often when there has been prolonged exposure to small doses of radiation, although it may also develop from an acute condition. Inflammation is not as much of a factor in the chronic condition, but there may be extremely dry skin, hair loss and damage to sebaceous and sweat glands. The condition may also lead to skin cancers.

TCM Treatment

Cooling Solution to Reduce Heat and Toxins

Make this solution for use on cool compresses to reduce Heat and
Toxins. Apply it for 20 minutes, twice a day.

100 mL distilled water (蒸馏水, zhēng liú shuǐ)

5 mL glycerine (*Symphytum officinalis*, 甘油, gān yóu)

1 mL carbolic acid (石炭酸, shí tàn suān)

10 g smithsonite, or calamine (*Smithsonitum*, 炉甘石, lú
gān shí)

5 g zinc oxide (氧化锌, yǎng huà xīn)

To the distilled water, add the glycerine, carbolic acid, smithsonite
and zinc oxide. Stir until the powders are dissolved. Chill for at
least 20 minutes before using. Store in the refrigerator.

Gold and Purple Massage Oil

Use this preparation to massage affected areas whenever needed.

15 g angelica root (*Rx. Angelica sinensis*, 当归, dāng guī)

10 g gromwell root (*Rx. Lithospermum*, 紫草, zǐ cǎo)

10 g coptis rhizome, golden seal or Chinese goldthread
root (*Rz. Coptidis*, 黄连, huáng lián—literally "yellow
links")

10 g amur cork tree bark (*Cx. Phellodendri*, 黄柏, huáng bò
or huáng bǎi)

10 g Chinese foxglove, raw (*Rx. Rehmanniae recens*, 生地
黄, shēng dì huáng)

10 g turmeric (*Rz. Curcumae longae*, 姜黄, jiāng huáng)

100 ml sesame oil (*Sesamum*, 麻油, má yóu)

120 g beeswax (*Cera alba*, 蜂蜡, fēng là)

In a ceramic, enamel or glass saucepan, combine the angelica
root, gromwell root, coptis rhizome, amur cork tree bark, Chinese
foxglove, turmeric and sesame oil. Heat until the herbs become

dark yellow. Pour the oil through a sieve to remove the herbs. While the oil is still hot, add the beeswax and stir until it has melted. Store the oil at room temperature.

对话 (duì huà)

Sandy: We are seeing fewer severe cases of radiodermatitis, and fewer cases altogether, because of improved radiation oncology protocols. It still does happen, because the radiation has to go through the skin to reach the tumours. We support these patients with topical corticosteroids, and we monitor them for subsequent skin cancers triggered by the radiation over the long term.

Xiaolan: We treat this localized dermatitis with different methods, and this is another area for potential collaboration between us. Together, we can help alleviate patient suffering with this very difficult disease.

ROSEOLA (Exanthem Subitum), 幼儿急疹 (yòu ér jí zhěn)

Exanthem subitum means sudden rash, and it is also known as roseola, baby measles or three-day fever. We see it mostly in babies under the age of two, since 90 per cent of infants are exposed to it before they reach that age. It is caused by two human herpes viruses, HHV-6 and HHV-7, sometimes called roseolovirus. The disease generally starts with a sudden high fever and even seizures, due to the sudden rise in body temperature. Many children appear normal during this first phase of the illness. When the child appears to be recovering, a red rash appears, usually on the trunk, then spreads to the legs and neck. Unlike measles, roseola does not spread to the face or cause eye problems. It is important to check on this disease, as its symptoms resemble those of more serious conditions, such as measles or even meningitis.

TCM Treatment

Little Angel Herbal Mineral Bath

Sponge-bathe the child with this infusion once a day.

- 20 g   sophora root (*Rx. Sophora,* 苦参, kǔ shēn)
- 20 g   Siberian cocklebur fruit (*Fr. Xanthium,* 苍耳, cāng ěr)
- 15 g   vaccaria (*Se. Vaccaria,* 王不留行, wáng bù liú xíng)
- 10 g   alum (*Potassium Aluminum Sulphate,* 明矾, míng fán)
- 2 L   water

In a ceramic, enamel or glass saucepan, combine all the ingredients. Let soak for 2 hours, then bring to a boil and simmer for 45 minutes. Pour through a sieve, reserving the liquid. Discard the pulp. Use the liquid to sponge-bathe the affected areas.

Mother's Milk Healing Tea for Roseola

If the condition is severe and the mother is still breastfeeding, she can drink this tea in addition to using the Little Angel Herbal Mineral Bath above. She should drink 250 mL in the morning and 250 mL in the evening.

- 20 g   gromwell root (*Rx. Lithospermum,* 紫草根, zǐ cǎo gēn)
- 15 g   Chinese foxglove, raw (*Rx. Rehmanniae recens,* 生地黄, shēng dì huáng)
- 15 g   hedyotis (*Hb. Oldenlandia,* 白花蛇舌草, bái huā shé shé cǎo)
- 15 g   root bark of shaggy-fruited dittany (*Cs. Dictamni,* 白鲜皮, bái xiān pí)
- 15 g   Chinese arborvitae twig and leaf (*Cacumen Biotae orientalis,* 侧柏叶, cè bó yè)
- 12 g   wild chrysanthemum (*Fl. Chrysanthemi indici,* 野菊花, yě jú huā)
- 12 g   *Saposhnikovia divaricata* root (*Rx. Ledebouriella,* 防风, fáng fēng)

3 g   licorice (*Rx. Glycyrrhizae,* 甘草, gān cǎo)

2 L   water

In a ceramic, enamel or glass saucepan, combine all the ingredients. Let soak for 2 hours, then bring to a boil and simmer for 45 minutes, or until reduced to 500 mL.

Healing Baby Paste for Roseola

Make this paste to apply to the lesions three times a day.

30 g   Chinese rhubarb root powder (*Rx. et Rz. Rhei,* 大黄粉, dà huáng fěn)

10 g   sulphur powder (硫黄粉, liú huáng fěn)

Water

Combine the powders with enough water to make a paste. Store in a sealed jar at room temperature.

Parents can massage the baby.

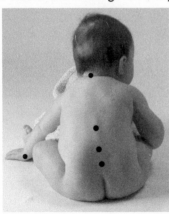 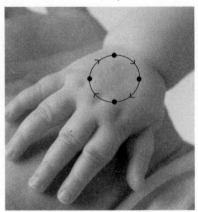

对话 (duì huà)

Sandy: Roseola is generally a mild viral infection. We recommend acetaminophen or non-steroidal anti-inflammatory drugs for fever control (although not ASA for children). However, because fewer people are getting their children immunized for measles, which can be serious, it is important to establish which condition it is. Like Xiaolan, I think that controlling fever in children is important to prevent seizures.

S

SHINGLES or Herpes Zoster, 带状疱疹 (dài zhuàng pàozhěn)

Shingles, also known as Herpes Zoster or Varicella Zoster, is actually caused by the same virus as chicken pox, which sometimes hibernates in nerve ganglions and re-emerges later in life (most commonly in people after the age of 50) in the form of acutely painful skin eruptions and nerve pain. Sometimes the severe nerve pain can persist long after the rash has healed.

TCM Treatment

See treatments for Varicella Zoster (Chicken Pox) on p. 198.

Western Treatment

In mild cases, Western medicine holds that the virus just needs to run its course, but in more severe cases—children, pregnant women or anyone under the age of 50—it is important to treat it in the first 48 to 72 hours. The treatment usually consists of antiviral drugs such as Acyclovir and pain medication as needed.

SKIN CANCER, 皮肤癌 (pí fū ái)

Skin cancer is a malignant growth on or in the skin. There are different types, and some are more virulent and problematic than others. They are the most commonly diagnosed cancers of all. With the exception of the deadly melanoma, death rates from skin cancers such as basal cell and squamous cell carcinomas are markedly lower than for other cancers. This may be in part because their origin in the epidermis, the top layer of skin, makes them visible from an early stage, improving the rate of diagnosis over internal cancers, which can be hard to detect at first. The vast majority of skin cancers are caused by excessive exposure to the sun. Patients who have had just one blistering sunburn have a 50 per cent greater chance of developing basal cell carcinoma.

Basal cell carcinomas (基底细胞癌, jī dǐ xì bāo ái), the most common form of skin cancer, are usually localized growths caused by excessive cumulative sun exposure over a lifetime; they are therefore far more common with advancing age. About 30 per cent of Caucasians develop a basal cell cancer within their lifetime. Eighty per cent of basal cell cancers are on the head or the neck. They first appear as shiny, pearly nodules or red patches like eczema. It can be difficult to distinguish basal cell carcinomas from other skin conditions such as acne scars, actinic elastosis or inflammations. Therefore it is essential to obtain a diagnosis—sometimes, though not always, through a biopsy. Usually, this can be done under a local anaesthetic in the dermatologist's office.

Squamous cell carcinomas (鳞状细胞癌, lín zhuàng xì bāo ái) are the second most common skin cancer after basal cell carcinomas. They can arise in many different organs, including the skin, lips, mouth, esophagus, urinary bladder, prostate, lungs, vagina and cervix. They are malignant tumours of the epithelium, which is the middle part of the epidermis, or the top layer of tissue in mucous tissues. They can begin with a small nodule. As it grows larger, the tissue in the centre of it dies and falls away; the nodule turns into a slow-growing ulcer. Unfortunately, this lesion can be asymptomatic, making this cancer harder to detect.

Tumours can bleed intermittently, especially on the lip. The edges may be hard and raised. This often occurs on sun-exposed areas such as the back of the hand, the scalp or the lip. Unlike basal cell carcinoma, squamous cell carcinomas often spread; this risk is higher in scar tissue, in mucous tissues such as the lower lips, and in patients with compromised or suppressed immune systems. About one-third of patients (often tobacco or alcohol users) metastasize before diagnosis. Human papilloma virus (HPV) has been associated with squamous cell carcinoma of the oropharynx, lung, finger and anogenital region.

Melanoma, the most serious of the skin cancers, causes three-quarters of all skin cancer deaths—about 48,000 people a year, according to the World Health Organization. Unfortunately, it is on the rise in general, but the highest increases are among teenage girls, the heaviest users of tanning salons. There is also speculation that additional factors may be at play: more relaxed standards of dress, which result in more skin being exposed to the sun, the thinning ozone layer, longer vacation time outdoors, and earlier sunscreen formulas that did not cover the UVA spectrum.

The melanocytes, the cells responsible for skin pigmentation, also protect the skin from sun damage. When you spend time in the sun or in a tanning salon, the melanocytes respond by making more melanin to protect the deeper layers of skin. This added colour provides the tanning that so many people enjoy. But it also increases the likelihood that the melanocytes will begin to mutate, or grow abnormally, and become cancerous.

Melanoma often appears as a change in the size, shape or colour of a mole anywhere on the body. But it can also appear as a new mole—in men, most often on the upper body, between the shoulders and hips or on the head and neck, and in women, most often on the lower legs. In dark-skinned people, melanoma most often appears under the fingernails or toenails, on the palms of the hands or on the soles of the feet. The chance of getting melanoma increases with age, but it is one of the most common cancers in young adults. It is more common among males, all Caucasians, particularly those who live in sunny climates, and those who use tanning salons.

It is extremely important to be aware of these changes on your body, as early diagnosis and treatment are closely linked to the chances of recovery.

TCM Treatment

As with all forms of cancer, the best treatment is collaborative between Western and TCM practitioners. The TCM approach will support the patient through the Western interventions with detoxifying and strength-building measures, as well as help to mitigate the side effects of difficult treatments such as chemotherapy, radiation and surgery. TCM will also help to handle scar tissue that results from surgery, radiation burns or other events.

With skin cancer, TCM will treat the lesions topically and use an infusion to support the patient's overall resistance to the disease. In the early stages of cancer, TCM seeks to clear the toxic Heat, which it holds responsible for the progression of cancer and for bringing on swelling, lumps, pain, fever, irritability, dry mouth and throat, constipation and other symptoms. The herbs used to counter these reactions will have a cooling effect and help to inhibit the growth of cancer cells.

TCM will also seek to supplement the Blood and dissipate Blood Stasis, which it holds responsible for helping cancer cells to embed in new areas and grow. Blood Stasis is associated with tumours, localized pain, a purplish tongue and skin, dry and rough skin, brittle nails and varicose veins. Stimulating blood flow and thinning the blood can help to shrink the tumour and inhibit the growth of its surrounding connective tissues.

Cancer patients need a range of support, including detoxification, balancing the body's systems to maximize the chances of recovery, and assistance to promote their peace of mind. TCM plays an auxiliary role, helping to not only mitigate the side effects of cancer treatment but also keep patients strong.

Cooling Analgesic Herbal Wash

This wash is also good for use on cold compresses for injuries such as soft-tissue injuries and headaches, but not where the skin is broken.

20 g   wild chrysanthemum (*Fl. Chrysanthemi indici,* 野菊花, yě jú huā)

20 g   garden burnet root (*Rx. Sanguisorbia,* 地榆, dì yú)

15 g   Chinese rhubarb (*Rx. et Rz. Rhei,* 大黄, dà huáng)

15 g   sophora root (*Rx. Sophora,* 苦参, kǔ shēn)

15 g   catmint (*Hb. Schizonepeta,* 荆芥, jīng jiè)

12 g   bur-reed rhizome, or scirpus (*Sparganium stoloniferum,* 三棱, sān léng)

12 g   zedoaria (*Curcuma zedoaria,* 莪术, é zhú)

10 g   burnt alum (*Potassium Aluminum Sulphate,* 烧明矾, shāo míng fán)

2 L   water

In a ceramic, enamel or glass saucepan, combine all the ingredients. Let soak for 2 hours, then bring to a boil and simmer for 45 minutes. Pour through a sieve, reserving the liquid. Discard the pulp. Use the liquid to sponge-bathe the affected areas as needed for pain.

Move-It Cool-It Tea

Drink 250 mL of this tea in the morning and 250 mL in the evening to support clearing the toxic Heat internally, supplement the Blood and dissipate Blood Stasis.

30 g   barbed skullcap (*Rx. Scutellariae barbata,* 半枝莲, bàn zhī lián)

20 g   glabrous greenbrier root (*Rz. Smilacis glabrae,* 土茯苓, tǔ fú ling)

15 g   hedyotis (*Hb. Oldenlandia,* 白花蛇舌草, bái huā shé shé cǎo)

15 g   tinospora root, or tulip bulb (*Tinospora sagittata,* 山慈姑, shān cí gū)

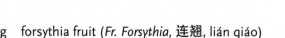

15 g   forsythia fruit (*Fr. Forsythia*, 连翘, lián qiáo)

12 g   ningpo figwort (*Rx. Scrophuloriae*, 玄参, xuán shēn)

12 g   red peony root (*Rx. Paeonia rubra*, 赤芍, chì sháo)

12 g   bur-reed rhizome, or scirpus (*Sparganium stoloniferum*, 三棱, sān léng)

12 g   zedoaria (*Curcuma zedoaria*, 莪术, é zhú)

12 g   salvia root (*Rx. Salvia*, 丹参, dān shēn)

6 g   licorice (*Rx. Glycyrrhizae*, 甘草, gān cǎo)

2 L   water

In a ceramic, enamel or glass saucepan, combine all the ingredients. Let soak for 2 hours, then bring to a boil and simmer for 45 minutes, or until reduced to 500 mL.

Tonic Balancing Tea

When the cancer reaches an advanced stage, it is vital to support the body as a whole and stimulate the appetite. Drink 250 mL of this tea in the morning and 250 mL in the evening to replenish the Blood and Qi, fortify the organs and rebalance the body's Yin and Yang.

20 g   astragalus (*Rx. Astragali*, 黄芪, huáng qí)

20 g   polygonati (*Rz. Polygonati*, 黄精, huáng jīng)

20 g   Chinese yam (*Rx. Dioscorea*, 山药, shān yào)

15 g   seeds of Job's tears, or coix (*Se. Coicis*, 薏苡仁, yì yǐ rén)

15 g   cinnamon twig, or cornelian cherry (*Cx. Cinnamomi*, 桂枝, guì zhī)

12 g   poria (*Poria*, 茯苓, fú líng)

12 g   angelica root (*Rx. Angelica sinensis*, 当归, dāng guī)

12 g   Szechuan lovage root (*Rz. Ligustici Wall.*, 川芎, chuān xiōng)

12 g   tangerine peel (*Citrus reticulata*, 陈皮, chén pí)

12 g   skin of the tree peony root, or moutan (*Cx. Moutan radicis rubra*, 牡丹皮, mǔ dān pí)

6 g   honey-fried licorice (*Rx. Glycyrrhizae preparata*, 炙甘
      草, zhì gān cǎo)
2 L   water

In a ceramic, enamel or glass saucepan, combine all the ingredients.
Let soak for 2 hours, then bring to a boil and simmer for 45 minutes,
or until reduced to 500 mL.

Herbal Mineral Root Wash
With melanoma patients, we wash the affected areas with this
solution.

20 g   Chinese rhubarb (*Rx. et Rz. Rhei*, 大黄, dà huáng)
20 g   sophora root (*Rx. Sophora*, 苦参, kǔ shēn)
20 g   garden burnet root (*Rx. Sanguisorbia*, 地榆, dì yú)
20 g   zedoaria (*Curcuma zedoaria*, 莪术, é zhú)
20 g   bur-reed rhizome, or scirpus (*Sparganium
       stoloniferum*, 三棱, sān léng)
15 g   wild chrysanthemum (*Fl. Chrysanthemi indici*, 野菊花,
       yě jú huā)
15 g   catmint (*Hb. Schizonepeta*, 荆芥, jīng jiè)
10 g   burnt alum (*Potassium Aluminum Sulphate*, 烧明矾,
       shāo míng fán)
2 L   water

In a ceramic, enamel or glass saucepan, combine all the ingredients.
Let soak for 2 hours, then bring to a boil and simmer for 45 minutes.
Pour through a sieve, reserving the liquid. Discard the pulp. Use the
liquid to sponge-bathe the affected areas as needed for pain.

Peace and Tranquility Tea
Melanoma patients should also drink this tea: 250 mL in the morning and 250 mL in the evening.

20 g   seeds of Job's tears, or coix (*Se. Coicis*, 薏苡仁, yì yǐ rén)

15 g	hedyotis (*Hb. Oldenlandia*, 白花蛇舌草, bái huā shé shé cǎo)
15 g	barbed skullcap (*Rx. Scutellariae barbata*, 半枝莲, bàn zhī lián)
15 g	honeysuckle flower (*Fl. Lonicera*, 金银花, jīn yín huā)
15 g	bupleurum (*Rx. Bupleuri*, 柴胡, chái hú)
12 g	salvia root (*Rx. Salvia*, 丹参, dān shēn)
12 g	gromwell root (*Rx. Lithospermum*, 紫草, zǐ cǎo)
12 g	indigo leaf (*Folium Daqingye*, 大青叶, dà qīng yè)
3 g	licorice (*Rx. Glycyrrhizae*, 甘草, gān cǎo)
2 L	water

In a ceramic, enamel or glass saucepan, combine all the ingredients. Let soak for 2 hours, then bring to a boil and simmer for 45 minutes, or until reduced to 500 mL.

对话 (duì huà)

Sandy: Melanoma treatment consists of early diagnosis and excision of the diseased tissues with margins of healthy tissue all around them. If it has spread beyond the skin, treatment involves drugs such as interferon-alpha (biologic therapy), some chemotherapy, which has limited effectiveness, and sometimes radiation in a small number of cases. There are vaccine trials going on to assist in the treatment of this lethal disease.

Basal cell carcinomas are usually easy to keep under control with surgery, radiation or a topical medication called imiquimod, and they do not tend to spread. The most common surgical treatment is curettage (scraping off). If the carcinoma recurs, it will be cut out with a small margin of the surrounding tissue.

Because squamous cell carcinomas metastasize more easily, they are usually excised immediately. If the cancer has metastasized, patients may need chemotherapy. Having either basal cell or squamous cell carcinomas constitutes a high risk factor of recurrence. Patients must be checked regularly, both at the original sites and all over their bodies.

Xiaolan: If a patient has a growth, something that scabs, bleeds or has a change in colour, I would immediately refer him or her to you, Sandy.

Sandy: This is a strength of Western medicine. Most skin cancers need to be cut out. But as I have come to know more about your practice, Xiaolan, I can see that you are able to do a great deal to support cancer patients through their journey—and probably prolong their lives.

What You Can Do for Skin Cancer
Prevention is key, especially with melanoma. Once it has metastasized, this disease is extremely dangerous. If you have one or more of the risk factors, you should be seeing a dermatologist yearly for skin checks. It is crucial to avoid the sun and to use sunscreen.

SLEEP, 睡觉 (shuì jiào)

The importance of getting enough sleep cannot be overemphasized. The human body heals only during sleep cycles (see page 245 for the specific Organ cycles of sleep). When patients are having trouble sleeping, I suggest meditation techniques and breathing exercises to achieve peace of mind, which facilitates sleep. I also give them acupuncture treatment.

TCM Treatment

Dreamland Tea
Drink 250 mL of this tea in the morning and 250 mL in the evening for two weeks. This recipe makes enough for one day's supply.

15 g   schisandra fruit (*Fr. Schisandra chinensis*, 五味子, wǔ wèi zǐ)

15 g   Chinese foxglove, raw (*Rx. Rehmanniae recens*, 生地黄, shēng dì huáng)

12 g   spiny date seed (*Se. Ziziphi spinosae*, 酸枣仁, suān zǎo rén)

12 g   angelica root (*Rx. Angelica sinensis*, 当归, dāng guī)

10 g   codonopsis (*Rx. Codonopsitis*, 党参, dǎng shēn)

 6 g   honey-fried licorice (*Rx. Glycyrrhizae preparata*, 炙甘草, zhì gān cǎo)

 1 L   water

In a ceramic, enamel or glass saucepan, combine all the ingredients. Let soak for 2 hours, then bring to a boil and simmer for 45 minutes, or until reduced to 500 mL.

SMOKING, 吸烟 (xī yān)

I do not recommend that my patients quit smoking "cold turkey" until we have balanced their bodies and they are feeling healthy enough that their urge to smoke diminishes. Then I use acupuncture and diet to help them quit.

TCM Treatment

Smokers tend to suffer disproportionately from dehydrated skin and premature aging and wrinkling. Use wash and herbal prescriptions according to the skin conditions, as listed throughout this book.

Liver Support Tea

If you are a smoker, drink 250 mL of this tea in the morning and 250 mL in the evening to cleanse and maintain your health.

25 g   kudzu root, or pueraria (*Rx. Pueraria*, 葛根, gé gēn)

15 g   white mulberry leaf (*Morus alba*, 桑叶, sāng yè)

15 g   Yedeon's violet or viola (*Hb. cum Radice Violae yedoensitis*, 紫花地丁, zǐ huā dì dīng)

12 g	Baikal skullcap (*Rx. Scutellariae*, 黄芩, huáng qín)
12 g	wild chrysanthemum (*Fl. Chrysanthemi indici*, 野菊花, yě jú huā)
12 g	honeysuckle flower (*Fl. Lonicera*, 金银花, jīn yín huā)
12 g	indigo root (*Rx. Indigo naturalis*, 青黛, qīng dài)
12 g	dandelion (*Hb. Tara*, 蒲公英, pú gōng yīng)
12 g	spirodela, or duckweed (*Spirodela polyrrhiza*, 浮萍, fú ping)
3 g	licorice (*Rx. Glycyrrhizae*, 甘草, gān cǎo)
2 L	water

In a ceramic, enamel or glass saucepan, combine all the ingredients. Let soak for 2 hours, then bring to a boil and simmer for 45 minutes, or until reduced to 500 mL.

对话 (duì huà)

Sandy: The best treatment is prevention. Teenage girls seem to respond more to the fear of premature aging than to the fear of cancer. I tell all my teenage patients that the way they treat their skin now—through sun exposure, drinking and smoking—will trigger premature aging in twenty years.

Xiaolan: I, too, tell all my patients not to smoke, especially during pregnancy and around surgical and other medical interventions.

SQUAMOUS CELL CARCINOMA

See Skin Cancer, page 170.

STRETCH MARKS (Striae), 妊娠纹 (rèn shēn wén)

As the skin on a woman's belly expands, sometimes very quickly during pregnancy, the dermis can be stretched to the breaking point. (Sudden weight gain or muscle building can have the same effect.) At first the resulting marks appear as reddish or purple lines, but over time they fade to a lighter colour. The areas affected feel soft to the touch and lose their elasticity. Stretch marks happen only where there is loss of support in the dermis, and most frequently in places where larger amounts of fat are stored, such as the belly near the navel, the breasts, the upper arms and underarms and thighs, hips and buttocks. Between 75 per cent and 90 per cent of women will develop at least some stretch marks during pregnancy.

TCM Treatment

Supple Skin Bath

20 g	dahurian angelica (*Rx. Angelica dahurica*, 白芷, bái zhǐ)
20 g	apricot seed (*Se. Pruni armeniacae*, 杏仁, xìng rén)
20 g	willow bark (*Cx. Vitis*, 白蔹, bái liǎn)
15 g	Chinese ground orchid (*Rz. Bletilla*, 白芨, bái jī)
10 g	licorice (*Rx. Glycyrrhizae*, 甘草, gān cǎo)
2 L	water

In a ceramic, enamel or glass saucepan, combine all the ingredients. Let soak for 2 hours, then bring to a boil and simmer for 45 minutes. Pour through a sieve, reserving the liquid. Discard the pulp. Use the liquid to sponge-bathe the affected areas once a day.

Restoration Massage Oil

Use this oil to massage the affected areas twice a day, after a shower.

20 g	angelica root (*Rx. Angelica sinensis*, 当归, dāng guī)
20 g	turmeric (*Rz. Curcumae longae*, 姜黄, jiāng huáng)
20 g	gromwell root (*Rx. Lithospermum*, 紫草根, zǐ cǎo gēn)
10 g	licorice (*Rx. Glycyrrhizae*, 甘草, gān cǎo)
300 mL	sesame oil (*Sesamum*, 麻油, má yóu)

2 g   borneol powder (*Dryobalanops aromatica or Blumea balsamifera*, 冰片粉, bīng piàn fěn)

2 g   calomel powder (*Calomelas*, 轻 粉, qīng fěn)

In a ceramic, enamel or glass saucepan, combine the angelica root, turmeric, gromwell root, licorice and sesame oil. Let soak for 7 days, then cook over low heat until the herbs turn yellow. Pour through a sieve, reserving the oil. Discard the herbs. To the reserved oil add the borneol powder and calomel powder, then combine.

对话 (duì huà)

Sandy: There are limited Western treatments for stretch marks, or striae, but some patients find that moisturizers that contain glycolic or lactic acids can help to thicken the skin and make it more resistant to stretching. Post-pregnancy laser surgery can reduce the discoloration. Fractional laser resurfacing offers some promise. It is a novel approach in which pulses of light create microscopic openings in the skin that can stimulate new collagen production. This treatment has the disadvantage of being expensive, without any guarantees that it will work. Patients who are very concerned about this sometimes see a plastic surgeon for a "tummy tuck" to get rid of excess skin. This is a radical way to get rid of stretch marks.

Xiaolan: Stretch marks are a purely cosmetic issue with no health consequences whatsoever. While my treatments can help soften or even eliminate them, I do not feel that patients should put themselves through the trauma of surgery for such a small matter.

What You Can Do for Stretch Marks

The more weight you gain, the more stretch marks you will have. Keeping a healthy weight can help avoid them.

SUNBURN, 晒伤 (shài shāng) or 日晒 疮 (rì shài chuāng—literally "sun exposure sore")

A little sun goes a long way, especially for children, who are most at risk of overexposure to the ultraviolet radiation that causes sunburn and skin cancer. The face, neck and limbs are most vulnerable to sunburn, as they are most likely to be exposed. Strong sunlight can even burn through thin clothing.

Sunburned skin tingles during exposure and becomes red two to twelve hours later. The skin can swell or appear smooth and shiny. The redness is at its peak twenty-four hours later, then fades over the next two to four days, sometimes peeling and darkening. Mild cases cause burning and stabbing pain. Severe cases can cause blisters, which subsequently dry up and form crusts, as well as fever, headache, nausea and general malaise.

Make sure to read the note on vitamin D in relation to sun exposure (page 201).

TCM Treatment for Sunburn in Babies and Children

Little Chrysanthemum Sunburn Wash for Children
Use this solution to sponge-bathe the child as needed.

30 g	Chinese rhubarb (*Rx. et Rz. Rhei,* 大黄, dà huáng)
30 g	busy knotweed (*Polygonum curpidatum,* 虎杖, hǔ zhàng)
20 g	pinellia (*Pinellia ternate,* 半夏, bàn xià)
20 g	wild chrysanthemum (*Fl. Chrysanthemi indici,* 野菊花, yě jú huā)
2 L	water
45 mL	vinegar

In a ceramic, enamel or glass saucepan, combine the Chinese rhubarb, busy knotweed, pinellia, wild chrysanthemum and water. Let soak for 2 hours, then bring to a boil and simmer for 30 minutes.

Pour through a sieve, reserving the liquid. Discard the pulp. Add the vinegar to the reserved liquid and combine. This wash can be stored in the refrigerator for one week.

Strong Fire Cooling Wash
Use this wash for a more severe sunburn. Sponge-bathe the child as needed.

20 g   dandelion (*Hb. Tara,* 蒲公英, pú gōng yīng)

15 g   honeysuckle flower (*Fl. Lonicera,* 金银花, jīn yín huā)

15 g   woody grass (*Rz. Imperatae,* 白茅根, bái máo gēn)

6 g   licorice (*Rx. Glycyrrhizae,* 甘草, gān cǎo)

2 L   water

In a ceramic, enamel or glass saucepan, combine all the ingredients. Soak for 2 hours, then bring to a boil and simmer for 30 minutes. This solution can be kept in the refrigerator for a week.

Calming Fire Treatment Powder
Apply this powder to the affected skin as needed.

30 g   plantain (*Hb. Plantaginis,* 车前草, chē qián cǎo)

20 g   asarum powder (*Asarum sieboldii,* 细辛粉, xì xīn fěn)

20 g   licorice powder (*Rx. Glycyrrhizae,* 甘草粉, gān cǎo fěn)

20 g   powdered green tea (*Camellia sinensis,* 绿茶, lǜ chá fěn)

Combine all the ingredients and store in a sealed jar at room temperature for use as needed.

Balancing and Nourishing Aloe-Honey Paste
This soothing paste is good for all ages, and works just as well for frostbite.

1   45-gram piece fresh aloe (*Aloe arborescens,* 芦荟, lú huì) or 15 mL aloe gel

15 mL   raw honey (*Mel,* 生蜂蜜, shēng fēng mì)

Place aloe and honey in a food processor and process until combined. Apply to the skin for half an hour, then rinse gently with clear, lukewarm water.

Egg-Yolk Oil Healing Paste for Severe Sunburn

For more severe sunburn, you may also prepare this paste, which uses an excellent traditional egg-yolk oil base. It is perfect for babies and everyone else.

- 10 g   amur cork tree bark powder (*Cx. Phellodendri*, 黄柏粉, huáng bǎi fěng)
- 10 g   honeysuckle flower powder (*Fl. Lonicera*, 金银花粉, jīn yín huā fěn)
- 10 g   Baikal skullcap powder (*Scutelleria*, 黄芩粉, huáng qín fěn)
- 5 g   realgar (*Realgar*, 雄黄粉, xióng huáng fěn)
    Egg-Yolk Oil (see recipe below)

Combine all the ingredients. Use this oil to gently massage the affected areas of the baby's skin.

Egg-Yolk Oil (蛋黄油, dàn huáng yóu)

- 5   hard-boiled eggs

Separate the yolks from the egg whites. Place the yolks in a saucepan over low heat and cook them slowly until they are dark yellow and the oil separates from the solids. Drain off the oil and reserve it to use as a base for various massage oils.

Parents may also massage the baby to relieve the pain from sunburn.

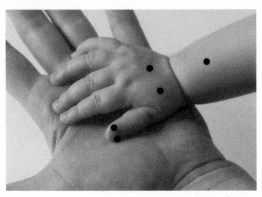

TCM Treatment for Sunburn in Adults
Use the Strong Fire Cooling Wash on page 184.

Cooling Sesame Paste

Twice a day, apply this paste to the affected areas for half an hour, then rinse off gently with clear, lukewarm water. Continue using the paste for as long as it's needed.

50 g   gypsum fibrosum powder (*Gypsum fibrosum*, 石膏粉, shí gāo fěn)

20 g   calcitum (*Calcitum*, 寒水石, hán shuǐ shí)

5 g   borneol powder (*Dryobalanops aromatica or Blumea balsamifera*, 冰片粉, bīng piàn fěn)

5 g   calomel powder (*Calomelas*, 轻 粉, qīng fěn)
       Sesame oil (*Sesamum*, 麻油, má yóu)

Combine the gypsum fibrosum powder, calcitum, borneol powder and calomel powder. Mix in enough sesame oil to make a paste.

Sun God Recovery Tea

Drink 250 mL of this tea in the morning and 250 mL in the evening.

20 g   Chinese foxglove, raw (*Rx. Rehmanniae recens*, 生地
        黄, shēng dì huáng)

15 g   honeysuckle flower (*Fl. Lonicera*, 金银花, jīn yín huā)

15 g   Chinese yam (*Rx. Dioscorea*, 山药, shān yào)

15 g   root bark of shaggy-fruited dittany (*Cs. Dictamni*, 白
        鲜皮, bái xiān pí)

12 g   forsythia fruit (*Fr. Forsythia*, 连翘, lián qiáo)

12 g   red peony root (*Rx. Paeonia rubra*, 赤芍, chì sháo)

12 g   wild chrysanthemum (*Fl. Chrysanthemi indici*, 野菊花,
        yě jú huā)

12 g   anemarrhena rhizome (*Anemarrhena asphodeloides*,
        知母, zhī mǔ—literally "know about mother")

12 g   lophatherum, or bamboo leaves (*Lophatherum gracile
        Brongniart*, 淡竹叶, dàn zhú yè)

12 g   prunella (*Spica prunellae*, 夏枯草, xià kū cǎo)

3 g   licorice (*Rx. Glycyrrhizae*, 甘草, gān cǎo)

2 L   water

In a ceramic, enamel or glass saucepan, combine all the ingredients. Let soak for 2 hours, then bring to a boil and simmer for 45 minutes, or until reduced to 500 mL.

PHOTO DAMAGE, 阳光损伤早期迹象 (rì guāng sǔn shāng zǎo qí jī xiàng)

Photo damage happens over time whether or not we intentionally expose the skin to the sun. It is the result of exposure to UVA or UVB rays, and the damage is at the cellular level, including the melanocytes, the cells that govern pigmentation. A full quarter of our lifetime exposure happens before the end of the teenage years. The signs of photo damage include wrinkling, uneven or "pebbly" skin, irregular pigmentation, red markings, rough or scaly patches, freckles, liver spots (solar lentigo) and age spots, thin or fragile skin, pre-cancerous lesions and skin cancer. Photo damage happens most frequently where the skin is most exposed to the sun. Areas that are rarely exposed to the sun, such as the buttocks and the inner upper arms, can provide a good example of what a person's undamaged skin is like.

The best treatment for photo damage is prevention of further damage, in the form of protective clothing, including wide-brimmed hats, and wide-spectrum sunscreen.

TCM Treatment
Purple Rejuvenation Massage Oil
This treatment will smooth the skin and reduce its roughness, as well as delay further damage. Twice a day, massage the affected areas with the oil until it penetrates.

20 g	amur cork tree bark (*Cx. Phellodendri*, 黄柏, huáng bò or huáng bǎi)
20 g	gromwell root (*Rx. Lithospermum*, 紫草根, zǐ cǎo gēn)
20 g	honeysuckle flower (*Fl. Lonicera*, 金银花, jīn yín huā)
15 g	dahurian angelica (*Rx. Angelica dahurica*, 白芷, bái zhǐ)
300 mL	sesame oil (*Sesamum*, 麻油, má yóu)
5 g	borneol powder (*Dryobalanops aromatica or Blumea balsamifera*, 冰片粉, bīng piàn fěn)

In a ceramic, enamel or glass saucepan, combine the amur cork tree bark, gromwell root, honeysuckle flower, dahurian angelica and sesame oil. Over low heat, cook the herbs slowly until they turn dark yellow. Pour the oil through a sieve, reserving the oil. Discard the herbs. To the reserved oil add the borneol powder and stir to combine.

对话 (duì huà)
Sandy: Topical retinol-A and glycolic acid are the main agents known to help reverse photo damage, but they do not perform

miracles. Chemical peels and micro-dermabrasion can remove layers of damaged skin, but the new skin revealed by these treatments is more vulnerable to the sun for a short time, and should be protected with a broad-spectrum sunscreen. The next level of intervention is intense pulsed light (IPL, or photofacials). This helps target redness and brown spots. IPL is a non-destructive laser. There are also fractional lasers that actually remove damaged skin.

There are also radio-frequency lasers that tighten the collagen in the skin. I have not invested in these machines because I am not convinced that their results are consistent, given the cost to the patient. But at the end of the day, I feel strongly that sunburn should be avoided absolutely and should never happen under normal circumstances to young children in the care of their parents. Acetaminophen will bring down the inflammation and a topical corticosteroid will help the skin recover more quickly. If the skin blisters or has open sores, compresses, cool baths and topical antibiotics will help soothe and prevent infection.

What You Can Do for Sunburn
This is a no-brainer. *Everyone* should wear a hat with a brim of at least eight centimetres, and protective clothing for outdoor activities. Avoid long periods of exposure to sunlight, especially from eleven in the morning to three in the afternoon, when the sun is strongest. Use a high-SPF-factor sunscreen with broad UVA and UVB protection. If you do get a sunburn, external medication can reduce pain and diminish the burning sensation. Deal with broken skin immediately to prevent secondary infection.

T

TINEA (Ringworm), 股癬 (gǔ xiǎn) or 硬币癬 (yìng bì xiǎn—literally "coin tinea")

In TCM, tinea is mainly the result of Wind, Damp, Heat and worms invading the skin. Damp-Heat pathogens are most likely to attack during the summer. Profuse sweating or moist skin can trigger the disease by combining with Heat in the skin. The infection can spread through contact with infected clothing, cats, dogs or other pets or soil.

This superficial infection appears on the smooth skin of the trunk and limbs, the feet, hands or groin, and on the face. It starts as red scaly areas that can progress to raised bumps called papules, which multiply and spread to form one or many clearly defined circular, semi-circular or concentric lesions. They heal from the centre out, with raised "active" edges; they are mildly to severely itchy.

TCM Treatment

Wash the lesions with acidic lukewarm water, which will help to kill the fungus. If lesions on smooth skin are dry and itchy, use liquid medication before applying the powdered form, and avoid ointments entirely if possible.

Soothing Vegetable Bath

Use this solution to sponge-bathe the affected areas once a day.

30 g	dried mung beans (*Phaseolus mungo*, 绿豆, lǜ dòu)
30 g	fresh ginger root (*Rz. Zingiberis*, 生姜根, shēng jiāng gēn)
15 g	houttuynia (*Hb. Houttuynia*, 鱼腥草, yú xīng cǎo)
10 g	seaweed (*Hb. Sargassii*, 海藻, hǎi zǎo)

2 L   water

10 g   sulphur (硫黄, liú huáng)

In a ceramic, enamel or glass saucepan, combine the mung beans, ginger root, houttuynia, seaweed and water. Let soak 2 hours, then bring to a boil and simmer for 30 minutes. Pour through a sieve, reserving the liquid. Discard the pulp. To the reserved liquid add the sulphur and stir to combine. This solution can be stored at room temperature.

Soothing Anti-itch Paste

Apply this paste to the lesions as needed.

30 g   green tea powder (*Camellia sinensis*, 绿茶粉, lǜ chá fěn)

30 g   honeysuckle flower powder (*Fl. Lonicera*, 金银花粉, jīn yín huā fěn)

20 g   dark plum powder (*Fr. Prunus mume*, 酸梅粉, suān méi fěn)

Sesame oil (*Sesamum*, 麻油, má yóu)

Combine the green tea powder, honeysuckle flower powder and dark plum powder with enough sesame oil to make a paste.

Parents may also massage a baby with tinea.

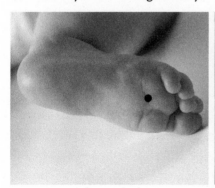 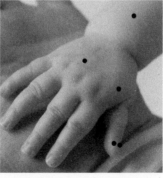

对话 (duì huà)

Sandy: These are superficial infections that do not internalize or become systemic, but they can affect the hair, the nails and any part of the skin. We use topical antifungals that kill the fungal organism (dermatophyte) that causes the infection. In some cases, especially long-standing ones, or where the nail bed or the hair follicles are affected, we may use an oral antifungal.

What You Can Do for Tinea

Avoid contact with towels or public baths used by infected patients. Do not touch infected pets.

THRUSH (Oral Candidiasis), 口腔念珠菌 (kǒu qiāng niàn zhū jūn) or 鹅口疮 (é kǒu chuāng—literally "goose-mouth sore")

In TCM, we see thrush in patients with Excess-Fire and with Deficiency-Fire. Damp-Heat in the Heart and Spleen is fairly common, especially among newborns. About 15 per cent of infants can develop thrush, usually as a result of an infection contracted while passing through the birth canal. Babies with thrush may drool, refuse to eat and suffer from irritability and low-grade fever.

Thrush looks like clotted milk: milky-white, velvety membranes most commonly on the tongue, the cheeks, the soft palate and the floor of the mouth. It causes burning hot pain and continues to develop. It can be serious in people with severely compromised immune systems.

Candida albicans is always present in a balanced mouth, but with thrush, it grows out of control and infect the mucous membranes. This most often happens when antibiotics kill the bacteria that keep the *Candida* under control, but it can also be the result of malnourishment or debilitation after a severe illness. It is common among cancer patients who have undergone harsh chemotherapy, which kills healthy cells along with the cancerous ones.

Thrush is classified either as acute or subacute, and is sometimes accompanied by a fever. When thrush arises in patients who have overused antibiotics, or who are simply debilitated, we often see Yin Deficiency–Fire patterns. It is much more common in undernourished infants, in those with diarrhea and renal failure, and patients undergoing long-term treatment with antibiotics, corticosteroids and immunosuppressants. It is important to understand that thrush is frequently a by-product of another disease. Treating this underlying primary condition is very important in curing or preventing thrush.

Hygiene is very important for everyone. In infants and children with thrush, mouths should be washed frequently with clean warm water or a weak saline solution. Breastfeeding mothers should always keep their breasts and their babies clean, and take care to sterilize their feeding implements. Never try to rub away the lesions, as this will cause bleeding and, potentially, infection.

Gentle Green Tea Mouthwash for Infants
Using a small piece of cotton or a swab, wash the infant's mouth twice a day with this infusion. Saline solution may also be used to wash the infant's mouth.

20 g   green tea (*Camellia sinensis,* 绿茶, lǜ chá)
10 g   licorice (*Rx. Glycyrrhizae,* 甘草, gān cǎo)
100 mL   filtered water

In a ceramic, enamel or glass saucepan, combine all the ingredients. Bring to a boil and simmer for 10 minutes. Pour through a sieve, reserving the liquid. Discard the pulp. Store the reserved liquid in the refrigerator.

Soothing and Nourishing Thrush Paste

If the condition worsens, apply this paste to the affected areas in the mouth twice a day.

> 50 g   dyer's woad powder (*Isatis tinctoria*, 大青叶粉, dà qīng yè fěn)
>
> Sesame oil (*Sesamum*, 麻油, má yóu)

Combine the dyer's woad powder with enough sesame oil to make a paste. Store the paste in a sealed jar at room temperature.

Parents may also massage the baby.

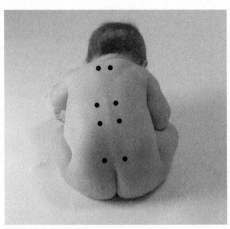

对话 (duì huà)

Sandy: In Western medicine, thrush happens more often in premature babies because the immune system is still developing. We only treat thrush if the baby is cranky and eating less. In these cases, we use a topical liquid antifungal. But if it is accompanied by a failure to thrive, this is a signal to look for other health problems, which may be more serious.

U

URTICARIA, 荨麻疹 (xún má zhěn) or 休眠丘疹 (xiū mián qiū zhěn—literally "dormant papules") or 风休眠丘疹 (fēng xiū mián qiū zhěn—Wind dormant papules)

Urticaria, also known as nettle rash or hives, is an acute reaction, sometimes provoked by an àllergen and sometimes difficult to explain, that causes bumps on the skin that can come and go quickly without leaving marks on the skin (hence the idea of Wind dormant papules). It can happen on any part of the body, at any age, with lesions that can be bright red, pink or milky white. Usually, there is intense itching. If the trigger for the reaction is external, such as a poisonous insect bite, it usually comes quickly and may leave just as quickly. If the cause is internal, such as acute stress, the condition can become chronic and recur.

TCM Treatment

Stop-the-Itch Wash

This bathing solution is suitable for babies and young children.

20 g	night kodo (*Solanacae*, 夜交藤, yè jiāo téng)
20 g	Siberian cocklebur fruit (*Fr. Xanthium*, 苍耳, cāng ěr)
20 g	shaggy-fruited dittany (*Cs. Dictamni*, 白鲜皮, bái xiān pí)
20 g	cnidium (*Se. Cnidium*, 蛇床子, shé chuáng zǐ)
20 g	sophora root (*Rx. Sophora*, 苦参, kǔ shēn)
15 g	puncture vine (*Fr. Tribulus terrestris*, 白蒺藜, bái jílí)
2 L	water

In a ceramic, enamel or glass saucepan, combine all the ingredients. Let soak for 2 hours, then bring to a boil and simmer for 30 minutes.

Pour through a sieve, reserving the liquid. Discard the pulp. Use the reserved liquid to sponge-bathe the affected areas as needed.

Purple Anti-itching Powder

    20 g   gypsum fibrosum powder (*Gypsum fibrosum*, 石膏粉, shí gāo fěn)

    20 g   indigo root powder (*Rx. Indigo naturalis*, 青黛 粉, qīng dài fěn)

    15 g   dahurian angelica powder (*Rx. Angelica dahurica*, 白芷粉, bái zhǐ fěn)

    15 g   realgar powder (*Realgar*, 雄黄粉, xióng huáng fěn)

    2 g   borneol powder (*Dryobalanops aromatica or Blumea balsamifera*, 冰片粉, bīng piàn fěn)

Combine all the ingredients and apply to the lesions as needed.

Massage the child's Meridians with Gold and Purple Massage Oil (see page 165) according to the drawing below.

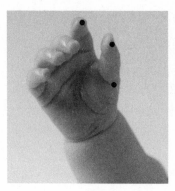
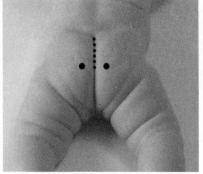

对话 (duì huà)

Sandy: Urticaria is very common, but 95 per cent of the time we never find out what triggered it. Many cases are acute and last several weeks, but if it lasts more than twelve weeks we consider it chronic. We treat the symptoms with antihistamines, sometimes combining them to achieve maximum effectiveness. If it moves to a chronic stage, we begin to look for chronic infections, thyroid irregularities, autoimmune diseases, food allergies or other explanations for the condition.

Xiaolan: TCM also finds it challenging to pinpoint the cause of urticaria. In China, it is sometimes triggered by parasites. In these instances, we destroy them.

Sandy: We rarely see urticaria caused by parasites in North America, although some of my patients have picked up a problem while travelling.

What You Can Do for Urticaria
If you can identify the cause, avoid ingesting it or contact with it. If you are susceptible to sudden allergic reactions, carry antihistamines or an EpiPen. Dress appropriately for the weather.

V

VARICELLA ZOSTER (Chicken Pox), 水痘 (shuǐ dòu—literally "water bean")

Since a chicken pox blister is oval-shaped like a bean and contains clear liquid, chicken pox is known in TCM as "water bean." Varicella is acute and highly infectious through airborne droplets. It is often epidemic in places where children gather, and they most often catch it between the ages of one and six. While having it early confers lifelong immunity, the virus does sometimes stay in the body and reactivate in later life as the painful condition called shingles (see page 170).

Varicella takes eleven to eighteen days to incubate, but when the chicken pox rash emerges, it comes quickly, starting with the trunk and spreading to the face, scalp and limbs. Since the rash can be very itchy, it can be acutely uncomfortable for children, particularly if it spreads to mucous tissues such as the mouth and the vagina. The blisters have a red halo and make little depressions in the skin after they burst. Patients are infectious from four days before the rash appears until there are crusts on all the lesions. Once the scabs are dry, they are not infectious.

TCM Treatment

Use the treatments given for Measles on pages 143 to 144.

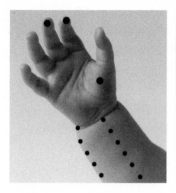
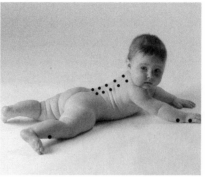

对话 (duì huà)

Sandy: This is a human viral infection. We treat the symptoms with fever-control agents and calamine lotion to control the itch. On rare occasions, we will consider an oral antiviral agent such as acyclovir, particularly in people with compromised immune systems or in adults with severe cases. When the sores are healing, we may use a topical antibiotic to prevent secondary infections and scarring.

What You Can Do for Chicken Pox

Oral hygiene is especially important during this illness. Avoid fatty, greasy or spicy food during the illness, which should not last longer than seven or eight days. The child's bedroom should be well ventilated, with plenty of light. Avoid drafts and control the fever. Isolate the child until the last spot has crusted, to protect others from infection. The child will want to scratch, but it is important not to do so in order to prevent scarring and infection. Keep the child's nails clipped and change clothes frequently. Use the Three Yellow Cooling Wash on page 80 to soothe the itching.

VARICOSE VEINS, 静脉曲张 (jìng mài qū zhāng)

There is a continuum between venous insufficiency, spider veins and varicose veins. Many people who never develop the gnarly "road maps" near the surface of the skin, which cause both health and cosmetic issues for women, do experience "heavy legs," a condition that arises due to poor circulation in the lower limbs. Varicose veins can be left alone unless they are causing pain and throbbing, or if the patient is greatly bothered by the cosmetic problem. Rarely, they can lead to other problems such as ulcers.

TCM Treatment
Three Yellow Cooling Bath
After soaking your legs in this bath, use a dry brush on the affected areas to stimulate circulation. Use circular motions and always brush in the direction of the heart.

30 g	sweetgum fruit (*Liquidambaris taiwaniana*, 路路通, lù lù tōng)
30 g	common clubmoss herb (*Hb. Lycopodii*, 伸筋草, shēn jīn cǎo)
20 g	amur cork tree bark (*Cx. Phellodendri*, 黄柏, huáng bǎi)
20 g	Chinese rhubarb (*Rx. et Rz. Rhei*, 大黄, dà huáng)
15 g	Baikal skullcap (*Rx. Scutellaria*, 黄芩, huáng qín)
5 L	water

In a ceramic, enamel or glass saucepan, combine all the ingredients. Let soak for 2 hours, then bring to a boil and simmer for 30 minutes. Wait until it has cooled enough to be comfortable for soaking your leg in it. Pour it into a container that allows you to soak your leg in the preparation for 20 minutes.

对话 (duì huà)
Sandy: Xiaolan, this is one area where Western medicine is interventionist. Women are often very disturbed by the appearance of varicose veins. For spider veins, we can inject a sclerosant or use new laser technologies to make them less visible. Venous insufficiency,

which can be associated with spider veins, can lead to brown pigmentation in the lower legs and to stasis eczema. The best treatment is prevention, through the use of compression stockings. With full-blown varicose veins with swelling and aching, I would refer the patient to a vascular surgeon to assess whether further treatment is appropriate to bring the condition under control.

Xiaolan: In the early stages of varicose veins, TCM techniques can slow their progress, but if they are severe, surgery is the best solution.

What You Can Do for Varicose Veins
If you are at risk for varicose veins, wear support stockings and exercise regularly.

VITAMIN D: The "Sunshine Vitamin"
If we all lived the way humans did thousands of years ago, in the ideal latitudes so that large amounts of skin are exposed to UVB rays for the right amount of time every day, we would never need to worry about vitamin D deficiency. This is because of the wonderful abilities of the human body to regulate itself. Exposure to the sun stimulates the skin to produce vitamin D, an essential contributor to health, and also destroys it if we have too much, so that the amount of the vitamin in our bodies is in balance. With just a few minutes of the right exposure, the skin is able to manufacture up to 20,000 IU of the vitamin. Unfortunately, this only happens under ideal conditions that few of us ever experience today: during a few hours around solar midday, in the right latitudes for UVB rays to reach the ground. Those of us who live outside these latitudes or in cities, stay mostly indoors, have darker skin, wear clothing that covers up most of our bodies or use sunscreen to block cancer-causing rays are all vulnerable to vitamin D deficiency. For example,

the deficiency is common even in sunny India, where many people have dark skin and stay out of the midday sun because it is so hot.

More and more research studies are showing the importance of sufficient levels of vitamin D in preventing a host of diseases. The Canadian Cancer Society and the Canadian Dermatological Association (CDA) now recommend 1,000 IU a day, particularly in winter. That is up significantly from the 400 IU recommended in the Canada Food Guide for decades. Many countries are reconsidering the official daily recommended dose as the benefits of vitamin D come to be recognized for musculoskeletal health and to assist in preventing more and more conditions, including cancers, heart disease, rickets and multiple sclerosis. People on heart medication should consult their doctors about appropriate vitamin D supplementation.

The CDA does not recommend increasing sun exposure or using tanning beds, because of the increased risk of skin cancer—and certainly, the use of artificial and risky techniques purely for cosmetic purposes is not compatible with TCM's philosophy of inner beauty. The use of supplements is safe and an excellent way to maintain levels of beneficial vitamin D while avoiding the risk of getting skin cancer.

W

WEIGHT GAIN, 体重增加 (tǐ zhòng zēng jiā)

The combination of abundantly available high-calorie foods and a sedentary lifestyle makes weight gain very common in Western society. More than half of North Americans are obese or overweight—a trend that puts them increasingly at risk of diabetes, heart disease, cancer, strokes, sleep apnea and a host of other ailments. Recent research has found that social networks play a surprisingly important role in weight gain. Spending time with overeaters, whether they are friends or relatives, greatly increases the chances that any individual will also gain weight.[*]

Weight gain may also be the result of developing tumours or other abnormal growths (something requiring medical attention), or an increase in muscle weight through strength training (more often a positive development). Repeated cycles of weight gain and loss will result in stretch marks (see page 180).

TCM Treatment

Whenever I see my patients carrying extra weight—especially around the abdomen—I worry about the additional Toxins that patients carry in those extra fat layers. I find that people often gain weight when they are emotionally or chemically imbalanced. We support patients in returning to a healthy weight by detoxifying the Liver, supporting the Spleen's digestive function and helping the Kidney to stop retaining water.

---

[*] Rob Stein, "Obesity Spreads in Social Circles as Trends Do, Study Indicates," *Washington Post* (2007-07-26): A01; also Nicholas A. Christakis and James H. Fowler, "The Spread of Obesity in a Large Social Network over 32 Years," *New England Journal of Medicine* 357 (4): 370–379.

Liver Detox Bath
To detoxify the Liver, sit in this bath for 20 minutes.

50 g	fresh ginger root (*Rz. Zingiberis*, 生姜根, shēng jiāng gēn)
30 g	isatis root (*Rx. Isatidis*, 板蓝根, bǎn lán gēn)
30 g	gromwell root (*Rx. Lithospermum*, 紫草, zǐ cǎo)
20 g	dandelion (*Hb. Tara*, 蒲公英, pú gōng yīng)
20 g	root bark of shaggy-fruited dittany (*Cs. Dictamni*, 白鲜皮, bái xiān pí)
2 L	water
250 mL	iodized salt

In a ceramic, enamel or glass saucepan, combine all the herbs and the water. Let soak for 2 hours, then bring to a boil and simmer for 30 minutes. Pour through a sieve, reserving the liquid. Discard the pulp. Add the reserved liquid along with the iodized salt to the bathwater.

WRINKLES (Rhytides), 皱纹 (zhòu wén)
The following treatments are intended to keep skin supple and help prevent premature wrinkles from forming—usually from over-exposure to the sun. I do not think it is possible or even desirable to prevent wrinkles altogether.

TCM Treatment
Phoenix Seafruit Wash

50 g	finely ground oyster shell (*Concha ostrea*, 牡蛎, mǔ lì)
20 g	houttuynia (*Hb. Houttuynia*, 鱼腥草, yú xīng cǎo—literally "fishy-smelling herb")
20 g	ground peach kernel (*Se. Persica*, 桃仁, táo rén)
2 L	water

In a ceramic, enamel or glass saucepan, combine all the ingredients. Let soak for 2 hours, then bring to a boil and simmer for 30 minutes. Pour through a sieve, reserving the liquid. Discard the pulp. Soak a towel with the reserved liquid and hold it to the face for 15 minutes. Rinse gently with clear, lukewarm water.

Fine-Grain Polishing Paste
Exfoliate the skin with this paste.

30 g giant typhonium rhizome powder (*Rz. Typhonii*, 白附子粉, bái fù zǐ fěn)

20 g dahurian angelica powder (*Rx. Angelica dahurica*, 白芷粉, bái zhǐ fěn)

20 g *Saposhnikovia divaricata* root powder (*Rx. Ledebouriella* , 防风 粉, fáng fēng fěn)

Raw honey (*Mel*, 生蜂蜜, shēng fēng mì)

Combine all the powders with enough honey to make a paste.

X

XEROSIS, 皮肤 皲裂 (pí fū jūn liè—literally "itchy, dry skin")

Many patients complain about chapped, dry, cracked skin on the feet, the hands and the lips—especially during cold winters, and especially as they age. TCM attributes this problem to external Cold, causing Blood Stasis and consequent loss of nourishment to the skin. The skin loses moisture with age, and as we get older, more and more of us suffer from dry, itchy skin—especially in cold weather and in buildings with forced-air heating. Many people refer to this condition as "winter itch," and it can really affect one's quality of life.

An extraordinary number of my aging patients suffer from itchy, dry skin, especially in late afternoon and at night. Sometimes there is a reason why the skin behaves in this way, such as when there is a reaction to radiation or chemotherapy treatment for cancer. But in many cases, there is no visible cause for very itchy, dry skin.

Patients find that their arms and legs itch for no obvious reason, and when the cycle of scratching begins, they cannot stop themselves. They scratch and scratch until they break the skin, and then they have embarked on an infernal cycle that never ends. The scratches become infected and the itching becomes worse. At this point, the condition may tip over into eczema (see page 115). Some of these patients take antihistamines every day of their lives to control the itching. Others, determined to break the cycle, cover up their limbs and sleep with gloves on until the urge to scratch subsides.

In TCM, these symptoms clearly indicate a Yin-Yang imbalance, particularly in the Kidney. Whereas in younger years, the Heat that surfaces to make the skin itchy is a manifestation of excess Yang, with age this becomes a "Hollow Heat" due to a Yin Deficiency that leaves too much active Yang to make mischief at the surface of the skin. This is why all the herbs used to treat itchy, dry skin at this stage of life focus on cleansing and balancing the Kidney.

TCM Treatment

Rejuvenating Foot and Hand Wash

For dry, itchy feet and hands, try this lovely wash.

30 g	hydnocarpus (*Se. Hydnocarpus*, 大枫子, dà fēng zǐ)
30 g	skin of wolfberry root, or lycium bark (*Rx. Lycium chinensis*, 地骨皮, dì gǔ pí)
20 g	dahurian angelica (*Rx. Angelica dahurica*, 白芷, bái zhǐ)
15 g	tangerine peel (*Citrus reticulata*, 陈皮, chén pí)
1 L	water

In a ceramic, enamel or glass saucepan, combine all the ingredients. Let soak for 2 hours, then bring to a boil and simmer for 30 minutes. Pour through a sieve, reserving the liquid. Use it to sponge-bathe the feet and hands twice a day. Store the solution at room temperature.

Rich Moisturizing Orchid Paste

Apply this paste to the face and cover with a warm towel, or use a facial steamer if you can. Leave it on for 15 minutes, then rinse gently with clear, lukewarm water.

50 g	calamine powder (*Smithsonitum*, 炉甘石粉, lú gān shí fěn)
30 g	puffball powder (*Lycoperdon bovoste*, 马勃粉, mǎ bó fěn)
30 g	dahurian angelica powder (*Rx. Angelica dahurica*, 白芷粉, bái zhǐ fěn)
30 g	Chinese ground orchid (*Rz. Bletilla*, 白芨粉, bái jī fěn)

10 g   camphor (*Cx. Cinnamomi camphora,* 樟脑粉, zhāng nǎo fěn)
Lard (猪油, zhū yóu) or sesame oil (*Sesamum,* 麻油, má yóu)

Combine the calamine powder, puffball powder, dahurian angelica powder, Chinese ground orchid and camphor with enough lard or sesame oil to make a paste. Store in a sealed jar.

Dry Lip Moisturizing Paste
Once a day, apply this paste to the lips for 15 minutes, then rinse gently with clear, lukewarm water.

50 g   Chinese yam powder (*Rx. Dioscorea,* 山药粉, shān yào fěn)
30 g   cinnamon bark powder (*Cx. Cinnamomi,* 肉桂粉, ròu guì fěn)
Water

Combine the Chinese yam powder and cinnamon bark powder with enough water to make a paste.

Use Gold and Purple Massage Oil (page 165) above for the hands and feet. Apply liberally.

对话 (duì huà)

Sandy: This problem is much more pervasive in cooler climates, among older patients, and in people with a genetic predisposition to skin conditions such as eczema or atopic dermatitis. I see many patients whose problems are either provoked or aggravated by products that they use to clean their clothes and their bodies, such as detergents, fabric softeners, body washes and soaps with fragrance, bubble baths, and so on. In children, I frequently find that stopping the use of bubble bath solves the problem. I advise these patients not to use soap over their whole bodies, but to reserve it for the groin and armpit areas.

While moisturizing the skin is important, I always tell my patients that what is key is not what is in the product, but rather what is not. I advise them to use fragrance-free products. Glycerine and ceramides are helpful ingredients. In extreme cases, look for humectins—elements that actually draw moisture into the skin—such as urea or lactic acid.

Y

YEAST INFECTIONS, 霉菌性阴道炎 (mei jun xing yin dao yan)

Some vaginal yeast infections can result from an imbalance in the body's flora—for example, caused by overuse of an antibiotic that does not discriminate among the pathogenic and useful fauna, especially in the mucous tissues of the gut and the vagina. European doctors routinely prescribe live-culture yogurt with antibiotics to counter this.

TCM Treatment

Fragrant Healing Bath

For vaginal yeast infections, use this sitz bath.

20 g	Chinese gentian (*Rx. Gentiana*, 龙胆草, lóng dǎn cǎo)
15 g	patchouli (*Hb. Agastache*, 藿香, huò xiāng)
15 g	cloves (*Fl. Carylphylli*, 丁香, dīng xiāng)
15 g	Chinese rhubarb (*Rx. et Rz. Rhei*, 大黄, dà huáng)
10 g	coptis rhizome *(Rz. Coptidis*, 黄连 huáng lián— literally "yellow links")
10 g	alum (*Potassium Aluminum Sulphate*, 明矾, míng fán)
10 g	peppermint (*Hb. Menthae*, 薄荷, bò hé)
2 L	water
2 g	borneol (*Dryobalanops aromatica* or *Blumea balsamifera*, 冰片, bīng piàn)

In a ceramic, enamel or glass saucepan, combine the Chinese gentian, patchouli, cloves, Chinese rhubarb, coptis rhizome, alum, peppermint and water. Let soak for 2 hours, then bring to a boil and simmer for 20 minutes. Pour it through a sieve, reserving the liquid. Discard the pulp. To the reserved liquid add the borneol. Pour into a basin and sit in the liquid for 20 minutes.

We also recommend topical use of Gold and Purple Massage Oil (see page 165), with the addition of 2 g each of realgar powder (*Realgar*, 雄黄粉, xióng huáng fěn) and borneol powder (*Dryobalanops aromatica* or *Blumea balsamifera*, 冰片粉, bīng piàn fěn).

对话 (duì huà)

Sandy: In my downtown Toronto practice, the most common fungal infections among teenagers are various forms of tinea (see page 190), often caught from a pet, or from a fellow human on the wrestling mat.

Although vaginal yeast infections are not uncommon among teenagers, I do not see them often, as they would be more likely to see their family doctor for them. I am always conscious of the risk of triggering a vaginal yeast infection when patients use antibiotics for skin conditions such as acne, and I encourage patients to eat yogurt with live cultures or to take natural probiotics while they are on the antibiotic.

Glossary of Chinese Medicinal Herbs

English	Latin	Characters	Pin-Yin
acanthopanax root bark	*Acanthopanax gracilistylus*	五加皮	wǔ jiā pí
adzuki bean	*Phaseolus angularis*	赤 小豆	chì xiǎo dòu
akebia caulis	*Akebia trifoliata*	木通	mù tōng
albizia bark	*Cortex albizziae*	合欢皮	hé huān pí
alisma	*Rz. Alismatic*	泽泻	zé xiè
aloe	*Aloe arborescens*	芦荟	lú huì
alum		明矾	míng fán
amber powder	*Succinum*	琥珀粉	hǔpò fěn
amur cork tree bark	*Cx. Phellodendri*	黄柏	huáng bǎi

English	Latin	Characters	Pin-Yin
amur cork tree bark powder	*Cx. Phellodendri*	黄柏 粉	huáng bǎi fěn
anemarrhena rhizome	*Rz. Anemarrhena asphodeloides*	知母	zhī mǔ
angelica root	*Rx. Angelica sinensis*	当归	dāng guī
apricot seed	*Se. Pruni armeniacae*	杏仁	xìng rén
apricot seed powder	*Se. Pruni armeniacae*	杏仁粉	xìng rén fěn
asarum or Chinese wild ginger	*Asarum sieboldii*	细辛	xì xīn
ass-hide glue	*Gelatinum asini*	阿胶	ē jiāo
astragalus	*Rx. Astragali*	黄芪	huáng qí
atractylodes	*Atractylodes lancea*	苍术	cāng zhú
Baikal skullcap	*Rx. Scutellaria*	黄芩	huáng qín

English	Latin	Characters	Pin-Yin
Baikal skullcap powder	Rx. Scutellaria	黄芩 粉	huáng qín fěn
barbed skullcap	Rx. Scutellaria Barbata	半枝莲	bàn zhī lián
beeswax	Cera alba	蜂蜡	fēng là
belvedere fruit	Fr. Kochia	地肤子	dì fū zǐ
betel nut	Areca catechu	槟榔	bīn láng
biota seed	Biota orientalis	侧柏	cè bó
bitter melons	Mormordica charantia	苦瓜	kǔ guā
black cohosh	Cimicifuga foetida	升麻	shēng má
black sesame seed	Sesamum indicum nigra	黑芝麻	hēi zhī ma
borax	Borax	硼砂	péng shā

English	Latin	Characters	Pin-Yin
borneol	Dryobalanops aromatica or Blumea balsamifera	冰片	bīng piàn
borneol powder	Dryobalanops aromatica or Blumea balsamifera	冰片粉	bīng piàn fěn
bupleurum	Rx. Bupleuri	柴胡	chái hú
bur-reed rhizome or scirpus	Sparganium stoloniferum	三棱	sān léng
burnt alum powder		烧明矾粉	shāo míng fán fěn
burnt gypsum fibrosum powder	Gypsum fibrosum	烧石膏粉	shāo shí gāo fěn
bushy knotweed	Rx. Polygoni cuspidati	虎扙	hǔ zhàng (literally "tiger's cane")
calcitum	Calcitum	寒水石	hán shuǐ shí
calomel	Calomelas	轻 粉	qīng fěn

English	Latin	Characters	Pin-Yin
camphor	*Cx. Cinnamomi camphora*	樟脑	zhāng nǎo
capillaris	*Artemisia capillaris*	茵陈	yīn chén
carbolic acid		石炭酸	shí tàn suān
castor bean	*Ricinus communis*	蓖麻籽	bì má zǐ
catmint	*Hb. Schizonepeta*	荆芥	jīng jiè
chaenomeles	*Fr. Chaenomeles*	木瓜	mù guā
chaulmoogra seeds or hydnocarpus	*Se. Hydnocarpus*	大枫子	dà fēng zǐ
chih-shih bitter orange	*Fr. Citri aurantii*	枳壳	zhǐ ké
Chinese arborvitae twig and leaf	*Cacumen Biotae orientalis*	侧柏叶	cè bó yè
Chinese black date	*Fr. Jujubae*	大枣	dà zǎo

English	Latin	Characters	Pin-Yin
Chinese caterpillar fungus	*Cordyceps sinensis*	冬虫夏草	dōng chóng xià cǎo
Chinese clematis root	*Rx. Clematidis*	威灵仙	wēi líng xiān
Chinese dodder seeds, cuscuta	*Se. Cuscutae*	菟丝子	tù sī zǐ
Chinese foxglove (raw)	*Rx. Rehmanniae recens*	生地黄	shēng dì huáng
Chinese foxglove (raw) powder	*Rx. Rehmanniae recens*	生地黄	shēng dì huáng fěn
Chinese foxglove root cooked in wine	*Rx. Rehmanniae conquitae*	熟地黄	shú dì huáng
Chinese gentian	*Rx. Gentiana*	龙胆草	lóng dǎn cǎo
Chinese ground orchid	*Rz. Bletilla*	白芨	bái jī
Chinese honey locust spine	*Sp. Gleditsiae*	皂角刺	zào jiǎo cì
Chinese pink dianthus	*Hb. Dianthi*	瞿麦	qú mài

English	Latin	Characters	Pin-Yin
Chinese rhubarb	Rx. et Rz. Rhei	大黄	dà huáng
Chinese rhubarb root powder	Rx. et Rz. Rhei	大黄粉	dà huáng fěn
Chinese yam	Rx. Dioscorea	山药	shān yào
cicada slough	Per. Cicadae	蝉蜕	chán tuì
cinnabar	Cinnabaris	朱砂	zhū shā
cinnamon bark	Cx. Cinnamomi	肉桂	ròu guì
cinnamon twig	Cx. Cinnamomi	桂枝	guì zhī
cloves	Fl. Carylphylli	丁香	dīng xiāng
cnidium	Se. Cnidium	蛇床子	shé chuáng zǐ
cocklebur fruit or xanthium	Fr. Xanthium	苍耳子	cāng ěr zǐ

English	Latin	Characters	Pin-Yin
codonopsis	Rx. Codonopsitis	党参	dǎng shēn
common clubmoss herb	Hb. Lycopodii	伸筋草	shēn jīn cǎo
coptis rhizome, goldenseal or Chinese goldthread root	Rz. Coptidis	黄连	huáng lián (literally "yellow links")
coriander	Coriandrum sativum	香菜	xiāng cài
cornelian cherry	Fr. Corni officinalis	山茱萸	shān zhū yú
dahurian angelica	Rx. Angelica dahurica	白芷	bái zhǐ
dahurian angelica powder	Rx. Angelica dahurica	白芷粉	bái zhǐ fěn
daikon radish	Raphanus sativus	萝卜	luó bo
dandelion	Hb. Tara	蒲公英	pú gōng yīng

English	Latin	Characters	Pin-Yin
Saposhnikovia divaricata root	Rx. *Ledebouriella*	防风	fáng fēng
dragon blood	*Sanguis draconis*	血竭	xuè jié
drynaria rhizome	Rz. *Drynaria fortunei*	骨碎补	gǔ suì bǔ
dwarf lily-turf or Japanese snake's beard	*Ophiopogon japanicus*	麦冬	mài dōng
dyer's woad	*Isatis tinctoria*	大青叶	dà qīng yè
dyer's woad powder	*Isatis tinctoria*	大青叶粉	dà qīng yè fěn
eclipta	*Hb. Eclipta*	旱莲草	hàn lián cǎo
egg-yolk oil		蛋黄油	dàn huáng yóu
ephedera stem	*Ephedra sinica*	麻黄根	má huáng gēn
evodia fruit	*Evodia rutaecarpa*	吴茱萸	wú zhū yú

English	Latin	Characters	Pin-Yin
fleeceflower root	Rx. Polygoni multiflori	何首乌	hé shǒu wū
forsythia fruit	Fr. Forsythia	连翘	lián qiáo
frankincense	Boswellia carterii	乳香	rǔ xiāng (literally "fragrant milk")
gallnut	Rhus chinensis	五倍子	wǔ bèi zǐ
garden burnet root powder	Rx. Sanguisorbia	地榆粉	dì yú fěn
gardenia	Fr. Gardeniae jasminoidis	栀子	zhī zǐ
giant typhonium rhizome	Rz. Typhonii	白附子	bái fù zǐ
dried ginger	Rz. Zingiberis	干姜	gān jiāng
fresh ginger root	Rz. Zingiberis	生姜根	shēng jiāng gēn

English	Latin	Characters	Pin-Yin
gingko nut	*Ginkgo biloba*	白果	bái guǒ
ginseng	*Panax ginseng*	人参	rén shēn
glabrous greenbrier root	*Rz. Smilacis glabrae*	土茯苓	tǔ fú líng
glycerine	*Symphytum officinalis*	甘油	gān yóu
green tea	*Camellia sinensis*	绿茶	lǜ chá
green tea powder	*Camellia sinensis*	绿茶粉	lǜ chá fěn
gromwell root	*Rx. Lithospermum*	紫草	zǐ cǎo
gromwell root oil or purple oil	*Rx. Lithospermum*	紫草油	zǐ cǎo yóu
ground beetle	*Eupolyphaga*	土鳖虫	tǔ biēchóng
gypsum fibrosum powder	*Gypsum fibrosum*	石膏粉	shí gāo fěn

English	Latin	Characters	Pin-Yin
hawthorn fruit	Fr. Crataegi	山楂	shān zhā
heydyotis or oldenlandia	Hedyotis diffusa or Goldenlandia diffusa	白花蛇舌草	bái huā shé shé cǎo (literally "white-patterned snake's tongue herb")
hedyotis or oldenlandia powder	Hb. Oldenlandia	白花蛇舌草粉	bái huā shé shé cǎo fěn (literally "white-patterned snake's tongue herb")
hirsute shiny bugleweed herb	Hb. Lycopi lucidi	泽兰	zé lán
raw honey	Mel	生蜂蜜	shēng fēng mì
honey-fried licorice	Rx. Glycyrrhizae preparata	炙甘草	zhì gān cǎo
honeysuckle flower	Fl. Lonicera	金银花	jīn yín huā

English	Latin	Characters	Pin-Yin
honeysuckle flower powder	Fl. Lonicera	金银花粉	jīn yín huā fěn
hornet nest	Polistes mandarinus	蜂房	fēng fáng
houttuynia	Hb. Houttuynia	鱼腥草	yú xīng cǎo (literally "fishy-smelling herb")
hypoglauca yam	Rz. Dioscoreae hypoglaucae	萆薢	bì xiè
indigo leaf	Folium Daqingye	大青叶	dà qīng yè
indigo root powder	Rx. Indigo naturalis	青黛 粉	qīng dài fěn
isatis root	Rx. Isatidis	板蓝根	bǎn lán gēn
Japanese climbing fern spore	Sp. Lygodii	海金沙	hǎi jīn shā
kan-sui root	Rx. Euphorbia kansui	甘遂	gān suì

English	Latin	Characters	Pin-Yin
kudzu root or pueraria	Rx. Pueraria	葛根	gé gēn
lard		猪油	zhū yóu
licorice	Rx. Glycyrrhizae	甘草	gān cǎo
lilac daphne	Fl. Genkwa	芫花	yuán huā
litharge or galena	Lithargyrum	密陀僧	mì tuó sēng
lophatherum (bamboo leaves)	Lophatherum gracile Brongniart	淡竹叶	dàn zhú yè
lotus leaf	Nelumbo nucifera	荷叶	hé yè
lotus seed	Se. Nelumbinis	莲子	liánzǐ
lycium fruit (goji berries)	Fr. Lycii chinensis	枸杞子	gǒu qǐ zǐ
magnolia bark	Cx. Magnoliae officinialis	厚朴	hòu pǔ

English	Latin	Characters	Pin-Yin
mat rush	*Juncus effusus*	灯心草	dēng xīn cǎo
mirabilite or Glauber's salt	*Mirabilitum*	芒硝	máng xiāo
mother-of-pearl shell	*Concha Con. Margaritifera*	珍珠母	zhēn zhū mǔ
motherwort herb	*Hb. Leonuri*	益母草	yì mǔ cǎo
mugwort leaf, or artemesia	*Artemesia argyi*	艾叶	ài yè
mulberry mistletoe stems or loranthus	*Viscum coloratum or Taxillus chinensis*	桑寄生	sāng jì shēng
mume fruit	*Fr. Prunus mume*	乌梅	wū méi
mung beans	*Phaseolus radiatus or Phaseolus mungo*	绿豆	lǜ dòu
mung bean powder	*Phaseolus radiatus or Phaseolus mungo*	绿豆粉	lǜ dòu fěn
myrrh	*Commiphora myrrha*	没药	mò yào

English	Latin	Characters	Pin-Yin
night kodo	Solanaceae	夜交藤	yè jiāo téng
ningpo figwort	Rx. Scrophuloriae	玄参	xuán shēn
notoginseng	Panax notoginseng	三七	sān qī
notopterygium root	Notopterygium incisum	羌活	qiāng huó
olive oil	Olea europaea	橄榄油	gǎn lǎn yóu
oyster shell	Concha ostrea	牡蛎	mǔ lì
pagoda tree flower	Rx. Sophora	槐花	huái huā
patchouli	Hb. Agastache	藿香	huò xiāng
peach kernel	Se. Persica	桃仁	táo rén
pearl powder	Con. Margarita	珍珠粉	zhēn zhū fěn

ENGLISH	LATIN	CHARACTERS	PIN-YIN
peppermint	Hb. Menthae	薄荷	bò he
peppermint oil	Hb. Menthae	薄荷油	bò he yóu
peppermint powder	Hb. Menthae	薄荷 粉	bò he fěn
pinellia rhizome	Pinellia ternate	半夏	bàn xià (literally "half summer")
plantain	Hb. Plantaginis	车前草	chē qián cǎo
plantain seeds	Se. Plantaginis	车前子	chē qián zǐ
platycodon	Platycodon grandiflorum	桔梗	jié gěng
dark plum powder	Fr. Prunus Mume	酸梅粉	suān méi fěn
poison ivy	Rhus radicans	毒漆藤	dú qī téng

English	Latin	Characters	Pin-Yin
poison oak	*Rhus diversiloba*	槲葉毒葛	hú yè dú gě
poison sumac	*Rhus vernix*	毒漆树	dú qī shù
polygonati	*Rz. Polygonati*	黄精	huáng jīng
pomegranate husk	*Punica granatum*	石榴皮	shí liu pí
poppy capsule	*Per. Papaveris somniferi*	罂粟壳	yīngsù ké
poria	*Poria*	茯苓	fú líng
privet fruit or ligustrum	*Fr. Ligustri lucidi*	女贞子	nǚ zhēn zǐ
prunella	*Spica prunellae*	夏枯草	xià kū cǎo
pseudolaric hibiscus bark	*Cx. Pseudolaricis*	土荆皮	tǔ jīng pí
psoralea fruit	*Fr. Psoralea*	补骨脂	bǔ gǔ zhī

ENGLISH	LATIN	CHARACTERS	PIN-YIN
puffball	Lycoperdon bovoste	马勃	mǎ bó
puncture vine	Fr. Tribulus terrestris	白蒺藜	bái jí lí
purslane	Portulaca oleracea	马齿苋	mǎ chǐ xiàn
realgar	Realgar	雄黄	xióng huáng
realgar powder	Realgar	雄黄粉	xióng huáng fěn
red carrots	Daucus carota Var. sativa	红胡萝卜	hóng hú luó bo
red garlic	Allium sativum rubra	红皮大蒜	hóng pí dà suàn
red peony root	Rx. Paeonia rubra	赤芍	chì sháo
rice paper pith or tetrapanax	Tetrapanax papyriferus	通草	tōng cǎo
rice sprout	Orzya sativa	谷芽	gǔ yá

English	Latin	Characters	Pin-Yin
root bark of shaggy-fruited dittany	Cs. Dictamni	白鲜皮	bái xiān pí (literally "white fresh bark")
root bark of shaggy-fruited dittany powder	Cs. Dictamni	白鲜皮粉	bái xiān pí fěn (literally "white fresh bark")
essential oil of rose	Rosa damascena	玫瑰精油	méi guī jīng yóu
safflower flower or carthamus	Fl. Carthemi	红花	hóng huā
salvia root	Rx. Salvia	丹参	dān shēn
sargentodoxa vine	Sargentodoxa cuneata	红藤	hóng téng
schisandra fruit	Fr. Schisandra chinensis	五味子	wǔ wèi zǐ
scouring rush or shave grass	Equisetum hiernale	木贼	mù zéi
seaweed	Hb. Sargassii	海藻	hǎi zǎo

English	Latin	Characters	Pin-Yin
seeds of Job's tears or coix	Se. Coicis	薏苡仁	yì yǐ rén
senecio or climbing groundsel	Senecio cineraria	千里光	qiān lǐ guāng
sesame oil	Sesamum	麻油	má yóu
smithsonite or calamine	Smithsonitum	炉甘石	lú gān shí
sophora root	Rx. Sophora	苦参	kǔ shēn
sophora root powder	Rx. Sophora	苦参 粉	kǔ shēn fěn
spiny date seed	Se. Ziziphi spinosae	酸枣仁	suān zǎo rén
spirodela or duckweed	Spirodela polyrrhiza	浮萍	fú píng
stalactite	Stalactitum	钟乳石	zhōng rǔ shí
stemona root	Rx. Stemona	百部	bǎi bù

ENGLISH	LATIN	CHARACTERS	PIN-YIN
stiff silkworm	*Bombyx batryticatus*	僵蚕	jiāng cán
suberect spatholobus stem	*Cs. Spathoboli*	鸡血藤	jī xuè téng
subprostrate root	*Sophora tonkineenis*	山豆根	shān dòu gēn
sulphur		硫黄	liú huáng
sulphur powder		硫黄粉	liú huáng fěn
sweetgum fruit	*Liquidambaris taiwaniana*	路路通	lù lù tōng
Szechuan lovage root	*Rz. Ligustici Wall.*	川芎	chuān xiōng
Szechuan pepper or zanthoxylum	*Fr. Zanthoxylii*	川椒	chuān jiāo
tail of Chinese angelica root	*Rx. Angelica sinensis*	当归尾	dāng guī wěi
talcum powder	*Talcum*	滑石粉	huá shí fěn

English	Latin	Characters	Pin-Yin
tall gastrodia tuber	Rz. Gastrodiae	天麻	tiān má
tangerine peel	Citrus reticulata	陈皮	chén pí
Thunberg fritillary bulb	Bo. Fritillariae thunbergii	浙贝母	zhè bèi mǔ
tinospora root (tulip bulb)	Tinospora sagittata	山慈姑	shān cí gū
skin of the tree peony root, moutan	Cx. Moutan radicis rubra	牡丹皮	mǔ dān pí
trichosanthes or snake gourd root	Rx. Trichosanthis	天花粉	tiān huā fěn (literally "heavenly flower powder")
turmeric	Rz. Curcumae longae	姜黄	jiāng huáng
umbrella polypora or zhuling	Sc. Polypori umbellati	猪苓	zhū líng
vaccaria or cow cockle	Se. Vaccariaie	王不留行	wáng bù liú xíng

English	Latin	Characters	Pin-Yin
distilled water		蒸馏水	zhēng liú shuǐ
water chestnut	Eleocharis dulcis	马蹄	mǎ tí
white arsenic	Gauri pasana	砒霜	pī shuāng
white atractylode root	Rx. Atractylodes alba	白术	bái zhú
white mulberry leaf	Morus alba	桑叶	sāng yè
white peony root	Rx. Paeonia alba	白芍	bái sháo
wild chrysanthemum	Fl. Chrysanthemi indici	野菊花	yě jú huā
wild tarragon or star of the south (jack-in-the-pulpit)	Artemisia dracunuculus	南星	nán xīng
willow bark	Cx. Vitis	白蔹	bái liǎn
skin of wolfberry root or lycium bark	Rx. Lycium chinensis	地骨皮	dì gǔ pí

English	Latin	Characters	Pin-Yin
woody grass	Rz. Imperatae	白茅根	bái máo gēn
Yedeon's violet, viola	Hb. cum Radice Violae yedoensitis	紫花地丁	zǐ huā dì dīng
zedoaria	Curcuma zedoaria	莪术	é zhú
zinc oxide		氧化锌	yǎng huà xīn

CHAPTER FIVE

STRESS AND ENERGY

He who hurries cannot walk with dignity.
—Chinese proverb

I will never forget my very first shift as the abdominal surgeon in the hospital emergency department in Kunming. I was just twenty-five years old, about half the age of the very experienced head nurse in charge. Our first case was a six-year-old boy who had fallen off a construction scaffold from very high up in a game of hide-and-seek gone terribly wrong. The child was in a coma, and I was summoned to come and examine him to determine whether or not he was suffering internal bleeding.

As I rushed into the room, I was acutely conscious of all eyes on me. Who was this new young doctor? The highly professional team watched me with eyes full of doubt. My face was burning, my heart was in my mouth and my hands were shaking—I knew this was a make-or-break moment for the rest of my career in that hospital. Had I been the chief surgeon, the nurses would already have started an intravenous solution and an oxygen mask for the patient, but instead they were awaiting my instructions. They wanted proof that I knew what I was doing before they would truly accept my leadership.

I quickly determined that nothing was broken and that there was neither internal bleeding nor obstruction in the boy's respiratory and digestive systems. There was no neurologist available, so I also had to determine whether or not there was bleeding in the head or leakage of spinal fluids. I found no evidence of either.

With shaking hands, I wrote out the orders: oxygen, intravenous and close monitoring. I told the nurses I would be back in an hour, and to call me immediately if the boy's situation deteriorated. From the moment I issued the orders, the doubt was dispelled and we all came together smoothly as a team.

I walked back to my office, feeling as if my neck were swollen because my heart had been in my mouth the whole time. I sank into my chair, feeling totally drained. But I had passed the test. Under incredible pressure, a little self-control and years of hard studying had helped me pull through.

Although this pressure to perform was very stressful, it was quite different from the stress that I see among my friends and patients. I had not been allowed to choose my profession. No one even asked about my hopes and dreams for my future. As teenagers on a collective farm in China, we were told that some of us would be allowed to pursue an education. While I was reluctant to compete with my friends for the privilege, I was desperate to study. I applied and was chosen.

With a father who worked in broadcasting and a mother who wrote beautifully, I had been attracted to journalism. I thought that I might capture the emotions and thoughts that others could not put into words for themselves. I was called to serve in a different way: I was told that I would be a doctor. After graduating from medical school, I was simply assigned to a hospital and sent to live in quarters attached to the institution. Like most Chinese people even today—although this is rapidly changing—I did not have to devote any time or energy to such issues as where to work, where to live, what colour to paint the walls or what kind of furniture to buy.

While I do not think this was an ideal situation, I also think that it probably saved me from experiencing some of the stress that I see among my friends and patients who are constantly bombarded with choices: where to go, what to do, what to buy, what to see, what to support, when to make time for family and friends, whether or when to have a child, how many children to have—the list is endless, the emotional strain significant.

Young adults starting out in the workforce—assuming huge responsibilities for the first time, starting a family, buying a house—are under enormous stress, which takes a toll on their minds and bodies. As they mature, they learn to take these things more in stride, but the workload rarely diminishes. I see the consequences in our patients.

Dr. Sandy Skotnicki referred Robert to me after treating him for acute, chronic and severe eczema, which was clearly exacerbated by workplace stress. In his first few weeks on the trading floor of a large financial institution—a job where the pressure is constantly high, with even higher peaks—he suffered from cysts on his face. In addition to the usual itching and scratching all over his body, severe blushing and sensations of heat and prickling, he had also developed hemorrhoids.

Sandy had been able to help him significantly with getting his acute attacks of eczema under control, using corticosteroids and antibiotics. But she felt that he needed more treatment. Robert had learned that his condition was telling him something: he needed to take care of himself, eat properly, get enough sleep and remember what was important in his life.

Robert had already articulated clearly that he was experiencing Heat in his body—anyone could see that just by looking at him. In TCM terms, I told him that it originated in excessive Yang energy in his Liver. I used acupuncture and herbs to clear his Liver Heat and restore and nourish his Lung Qi. While Robert may always need help from time to time when the condition flares up again, I have been able to help him

For descriptions of eczema, dermatitis and other skin conditions linked to stress, as well as recipes for herbal formulas for topical and internal use, see pages 77–212.

with prevention and ongoing management of his overall health. So far, his condition is in remission and he is doing very well.

Sandy and I have been interested in finding more opportunities to bring together our knowledge of TCM and Western medicine to support our patients. Doris, a patient of Sandy's for many years, provided another opening. She had developed stubborn and chronic psoriasis while experiencing constant pressure from her aging parents. They called her every day and demanded that she devote her free time to caring for them.

Doris had not responded to the best Western drugs and only modestly to light therapy. Because she could not afford the more expensive biologic treatments that might have been better for her, Sandy started Doris on Soriatane, an oral medication that sometimes works. The highest dose was having some effect but was also triggering hair loss.

For a description of psoriasis and recipes for herbal remedies for both topical and internal use, see page 156.

A reduced dose successfully shrunk the lesions from 50 per cent to 20 per cent coverage of her body, but further progress was stubbornly difficult to achieve.

Sandy referred her to me. I treated her very differently from Alice (see page 10), although her diagnosis would be identical in Western medicine. While Alice was a small, slender person with acute psoriasis, Doris is slightly overweight and has had the disease for a long time. The chronic nature of her condition had depleted her so much that I did not attempt any detoxification but started her on herbs to support her Kidney Yang energy. Doris continues on the Soriatane, but the collaboration between Sandy and me seems to have improved her condition greatly. She is recovering, has far fewer lesions on her legs and is in much better spirits than she has been for many years.

In Doris's case, there was clearly an emotional dimension to her illness. This is an area where Western perceptions are very different from those in Chinese society. Chinese people are still very much influenced by both Confucianism and Taoism. Confucianism specifies codes of conduct and places a high priority on social harmony, achieved through a deep understanding of everyone's roles and responsibilities toward family and others. Harmony requires the restraint of emotions, conformity and compliance and subjugation to authority.

> If there is beauty in character, there will be harmony in the home.
> If there is harmony in the home, there will be order in the nation.
> If there is order in the nation, there will be peace in the world.
> —*Chinese proverb*

Taoism adds to the Confucian ideals of emotional calm and conformity an emphasis on the mystical elements of human nature. The fear of losing "face" or dignity through "wrongdoing" is also a powerful cultural determinant, as Chinese people are very concerned about not bringing shame on themselves and their families.

This explains why Chinese people are restrained in expressing their emotions and concerned about overall group harmony. They tend to associate emotional difficulties with physiological imbalances. If a feeling or an emotion is a body disorder, then it follows that there is little need to "work through" it in a psychological process. How Chinese people deal with their emotions and live their lives is chiefly governed by not having an ingrained cultural notion of personal choice, and having a habit of subordinating their individual needs to those of the family, group or society in general. The comparatively lower stress may help to explain why Chinese women have the lowest rates of breast cancer in the world, while Western women have the highest, although diet, lifestyle, environment and other factors are also important, of course. Among my patients, I see so many cases where stress has blocked the free flow of Qi and created an imbalance that threatens a patient's overall health. Sometimes the causes are immediate and obvious, as they were with Robert. In other patients, they can be the result of a lifetime of accumulated demands on the body. This was definitely the case with Sandrine, the mother of one of my patients. Her daughter had been urging her to travel to my clinic from her home in another city for years, but it was only when her condition became unbearable that she decided to come. By then, years of depletion of her Qi had caught up with her.

OVERLY FREQUENT PREGNANCIES AND THE DEPLETION OF ESSENCE

Every time a woman produces a baby, she spends nine months giving of her own Essence, from all the tissues in her body, to "manufacture" that baby. This process is extremely demanding and requires proper care and rest to recover. Overly frequent pregnancies will deplete a woman's Essence and shorten her lifespan, especially if she never experiences a Golden Month as Chinese women do.

By the time she travelled to see me, Sandrine had endured more than five decades of severe skin problems. She had tried every kind of professional she could imagine—and a few quacks along the way. A long series of dermatologists had given her increasingly stronger prescriptions for steroid creams that no longer worked at any dosage. Much of her skin was as thin and brittle as rice paper.

Although she was reduced to skin and bones, I could see that she was a woman of intelligence and grace, with a lively wit that flickered through her exhaustion and pain. Nine pregnancies without adequate recovery time had depleted her Qi and Blood to the point where she had no resilience at all. She was fragile and in the thrall of severe allergic reactions: swollen eyes, constant itching and pain. Her face was hot and fiery to the touch, and her feet were icy cold—classic symptoms of a severe Yin-Yang imbalance.

After feeling her pulse and looking at her tongue, I joked with her: "You are an unselfish mother: you have given all your Essence to your children. Now we need to put your assets back where they belong—inside you!"

Her eyelids were so inflamed that I could not even put an ice pack directly on them. I transferred cold from the ice pack to my finger and then to her eyelids. I also began to rub a soothing cream gently into her damaged skin. Immediately, she began to relax. She told me, to my surprise, that in all those decades of skin problems, no doctor or therapist had ever actually touched her skin. In addition to her other symptoms, she was suffering from "skin-hunger"—the need to be touched. We see this frequently, especially in older patients.

Sandrine stayed with her daughter in Toronto for a week. During this time, we treated her every day—not only with our entire TCM arsenal, to nourish her and get her Qi flowing and her Blood nourished, but also with a Western technique. Every day of that week, she received an intravenous high-dosage Myers' cocktail of B and C vitamins and minerals. By the end of the week, when we sent her home with a good supply of herbs, she could not believe how much progress she had made in just seven days.

She was able to face daylight without dark sunglasses. The unbearably powerful itching around her eyes and on several other parts of her body had subsided completely, and her skin had begun to regain its moisture and suppleness. She called her daughters back home and told them that in the short time she had been away from them, she had gone "from hell to heaven."

> Nature, time and patience are the three great physicians.
> —*Chinese proverb*

After her week in our clinic, Sandrine slept like a baby for the first time in months, free of itching and pain, and she continued to sleep well after her return home. At first, her symptoms appeared to be gone altogether. But Sandrine is one of those patients for whom patience is not a strong suit. In addition, she has a large family and many obligations.

As soon as she felt better, she began offering to help family members in other cities and travelling extensively. From time to time, her condition flared with fatigue and strong emotions. If Sandrine wants to recover completely, she will have to give her Essence time to renew itself.

THE IMPORTANCE OF SLEEP

With Sandrine, sleep deprivation caused by the unbearable itching and pain had greatly aggravated the depletion of her Qi and Blood. This is a distressingly common problem in the West.

I am constantly disturbed to see how little my patients sleep. Many of them work far too long hours and rest far too few. It is impossible to be in good health without adequate sleep. In TCM, each Organ system has its time and place in the daily cycle for healing and replenishment. If you miss this window, you are depleting the energy of that Organ. The diagram below lays out this cycle.

Each Organ has a two-hour time period in the day when the energy flow is at its peak in its Meridian. The energy flows in a clockwise cycle through the Meridians, and it is important to pay attention to this rhythm. Insomnia at a specific time every night can be a sign of trouble in that particular Organ.

Adequate sleep is also related to depression and mental health,

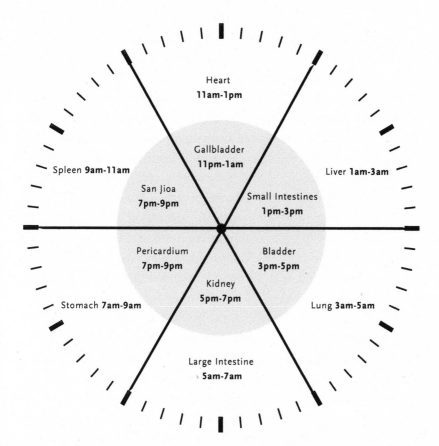

the spirit energy that is intimately linked to the Organ energy cycles. A TCM practitioner can detect problems in these areas almost instantly through the appearance of the patient's tongue and the quality, rhythm and speed of the pulses. Unlike in the West, where such skills were once common but have now been allowed to wither because of the total dependence on technology and sophisticated testing, TCM practitioners still use their own senses to help them make a diagnosis. I have a particularly sharp nose.

When I first came into the room where Sally was waiting for me, I could already smell the odour of her feet. She was a scrupulously clean person, and yet this smell clung to her body like a cloud around her, causing her considerable distress. She was embarrassed to raise the subject with me, and yet she knew that she needed help. She need not have felt this way: I was familiar with this strong and unpleasant smell, and knew it to be a sign of the presence of Liver Toxins, weakness of Heart Qi and vitamin deficiency, rather than a lack of hygiene.

For a description of fungal skin conditions and recipes for herbal remedies, see pages 123 and 210.

Sally was a senior executive with enormous responsibilities. She had developed psoriasis on her body and a fungus on her feet. She was sleeping only three hours a night because of her massive workload. In order to remain alert, she was chain-smoking and drinking seven cups of coffee a day. This, in turn, was driving up the acidity in her body to an unhealthy extreme. She had a history of manic depression and had survived three mental breakdowns. Now, again, she could feel the dark dogs of depression running close behind her, and she was determined to seek help rather than succumb once again.

A person whose heart is not content
is like a snake which tries to swallow an elephant.
—*Chinese proverb*

It took almost a year of weekly treatments to bring Sally back from the brink of this black hole. She stopped smoking and cut back her coffee consumption to one cup a day. On a healthy diet with abundant fresh vegetables, she also lost weight. She managed to change her lifestyle to get seven hours of sleep a night. Gradually, her depression began to lift. And to her surprise, the malodorous feet—something she had thought of as an incurable lifelong condition—cleared up within the year, as did her psoriasis.

Sally's case is a classic example of the ways in which TCM can provide holistic support to a person's health as she takes responsibility for her own lifestyle and choices. You would think that no one would understand the importance of a healthy lifestyle better than physicians themselves. But in fact, they are often the worst patients—perhaps because the daily stress of saving lives and caring for patients blinds them to their own state of health.

One day, I was having dinner with Daniel, one of my closest friends and a fellow practitioner. Like all doctors, he worked too hard, and in his case, his focus was strictly on his patients and not on his own needs as well. As we sat down to dinner, it soon became difficult to concentrate on our conversation. His breathing was shallow and rough, and I immediately became very concerned about the state of his heart. I knew he had a history of heart disease, and I knew that he operated at a constant and extremely high level of stress.

I asked him to show me his ankles and I insisted on taking his pulse. He laughed and said that I was overreacting; he simply wanted to enjoy our dinner. I insisted—I could not possibly have enjoyed the conversation while I was so concerned about him. His pulse was very irregular, and his ankles were swollen. Now I was alarmed. I made him promise to call his cardiologist in the morning. As it turned out, it took him five days to get to the cardiologist's office—but he was just in time. He lost consciousness in the waiting room and had to be rushed to hospital for an emergency intervention. One valve of his heart had completely given out.

How could my friend, a trained health practitioner, be so tone-deaf to the signals of his own body? As I have learned, it is possible for anyone to find that they are not listening to their body. This tone-deafness is particularly noticeable among my patients who are the most obsessed with their physical fitness.

I see a staggering number of injuries among patients who have spent years doing high-impact aerobics or marathon running. There is something about the pounding intensity of these sports that is very hard on bodies, and particularly on joints and bones. One particularly insidious injury is a cracked tailbone, which can be almost impossible to repair and can be a terribly intense source of pain. While it is more often seen in advanced old age, when osteoporosis sets in, severe symptoms have become much more common among vigorous middle-aged people who have misused their bodies and driven themselves into the ground with unnecessary exertion, such as frequent high-impact aerobics or obsessive running.

We all know that exercise is important; we all know that moving the body to keep the Qi flowing is a part of good health. But we need to remember that our bodies have limits— and we need to listen before it is too late. Although Western doctors often tell these patients that there is nothing to be done except to live on strong narcotic painkillers, TCM can often help in gentler and less invasive ways. Even though these patients' injuries cannot be reversed, TCM can alleviate their pain and their symptoms through the use of acupuncture, tui na and herbs, activating their own bodies' healing abilities as much as possible.

I sometimes ask these patients why they drive themselves so relentlessly. What I often find is that they have identified themselves too much with something that is not their Essence: their "perfect" bodies, their jobs, their status, their money, their model families—in short, their egos. Whatever it is, most often it masks their fear of dying. I tell all my patients: a healthy balance and moderation are key to good health and inner beauty.

It is just as important to get enough exercise as to avoid over-exertion. Extended periods of inactivity make Qi and Blood sluggish, and can lead to a Spleen Qi Deficiency. This can result in unpleasant symptoms such as cravings for sweets, weight gain, loose stools, excessive menstrual bleeding and muscle spasms.

It is important to balance the amounts of rest and activity so that we are not too sedentary, but also to avoid exertion that is too demanding and draining. Healthy sleep practices are also vital to this balance. Even people who appear to have the healthiest of lifestyles can fall into the trap of forgetting about the need for balance.

Tessie was a personal trainer with a sunny disposition, a happy marriage and a devoted family. Every morning, she jogged from her home down to the gym where she met her clients. Before she did her first hour of training, she would already have done a one-hour run. She would then train several clients for an hour each, before running back home.

There did not seem to be an ounce of fat on Tessie's body. She loved playing with her five-year-old daughter and longed for another child, but all her efforts to conceive again had led to failure. Such continuous strenuous exercise can exhaust Qi and Blood and lead to disharmony in the body. In women of child-bearing age, it often stops their Heavenly Water. When she came to see me, it had been months since Tessie had experienced a normal menstrual period. The first thing I said to her was: "Get a subway pass, Tessie! You don't need to run all the time—and you need a little fat to have normal periods. If you want to get pregnant, you'll have to exercise less. Moderation is the key."

Tessie was very surprised. She loved running and it had never occurred to her that something she enjoyed and did naturally could be harmful in excessive doses. It took almost six months of TCM treatments to bring her periods back to normal. Nine months later, she gave birth to a beautiful, healthy boy—one of many such stories with a happy ending in our clinic.

CHAPTER SIX

NUTRITION AND LIFESTYLE

*One should be just as careful in
choosing one's pleasures as in avoiding calamities.*
—Chinese proverb

In TCM, your body is your temple. This is what I always tell patients. If you can come to understand the direct link between the way you treat your body and your general state of health, you will have laid the foundation for a happy, balanced life and inner and outer beauty. It sounds easy, but it is not. Everywhere in the world, even among the best-educated people, the rates of obesity are skyrocketing—and children are not exempt, which is a cause for grave concern.

In many societies, but particularly in North America, we are beginning to see children and adolescents developing diseases that we have long thought of as the problems of old age: diabetes, heart disease and strokes, for example. Similarly, we are now seeing deadly melanomas in much younger patients, simply because of the popularity of tanning salons, which expose skin to dangerous levels of ultraviolet radiation. This is why governments are now beginning to ban access to tanning salons for those under the age of eighteen.

If you asked the average adolescent anywhere about whether they have ever thought about dying of melanoma, you would no doubt find yourself confronted with a blank stare. Most adolescents seem convinced that no harm will ever come to them. They are far more likely than adults to have unprotected sex and to contract unpleasant sexually transmitted diseases. The beauty of innocence that is the legacy of childhood can last for a long time, but it can also be brutally derailed.

> Medicine can only cure curable disease, and then not always.
> —*Chinese proverb*

I see many young patients for whom preventive counselling comes too late: for example, they may have to live with herpes for the rest of their lives. All I can do is soothe the symptoms and teach them to manage the disease intelligently. Since the virus re-emerges along the sensory nerve paths, lifestyle becomes important in disease management. I tell my young patients that they are at higher risk of painful flare-ups if they drink to excess, do not sleep enough or otherwise abuse their bodies. Having to tell a new-found love about this condition is a true test of maturity and integrity—and a painful life lesson for many of my young patients.

Teenaged girls are also highly vulnerable to vaginal yeast infections as they become sexually active, and to nail infections as they cover their nails with acrylic or other impermeable materials. The practice of covering natural nails with false ones that do not breathe, for years on end, often results in fungal infections of the nails. Over time, the nail bed becomes soft and vulnerable to these invasions. Teaching adolescents to care for the health and balance of their bodies begins by instilling in them from earliest childhood an understanding and respect for their inner beauty, which radiates with good health and does not require the addition of toxic chemicals and unhealthy procedures.

ILLNESS BY MOUTH, 病从口入 *(bìng cóng kǒu rù)*

The old Chinese proverb, "Illness comes in by mouth; ills come out by it," shows that for thousands of years, humans have understood that we abuse our bodies through what we ingest. Overeating, drinking alcohol and smoking are among the most prevalent causes of illness and death in the world. And obsessive under-consumption is as dangerous as overconsumption, particularly in diseases such as anorexia nervosa. What and how much we choose to ingest, important lifestyle practices that we will look at briefly in this chapter, can destroy both inner and outer beauty.

Binge Drinking, 酗酒 *(xù jiǔ)*

A cold beer on a hot day, a glass of fine wine with a good meal, a late-night whisky by a comforting fire—these are all pleasures that many people enjoy, and they form an important part of the social and cultural code in many countries around the world. There is also some research showing that moderate consumption of red wine and other forms of alcohol can have a positive effect on the heart and on blood pressure.

Excessive consumption of alcohol, however, is closely linked to ill health, tragedy and early death: drunk-driving accidents, broken relationships and cirrhosis of the liver can be the result. It is often easy to distinguish a heavy drinker from others, because alcohol also takes its toll on the most visible part of our bodies: the skin.

> A red-nosed man may be a teetotaller,
> but will find no one to believe it.
> —*Chinese proverb*

Alcohol is a vasodilator—that is, it provokes a chemical reaction that enlarges the blood vessels. When this happens repeatedly to the tiny capillaries in the face, they can become more prominent or burst, a condition known as acne rosacea. Alcohol also destroys the vitamin A supply the body needs to maintain healthy, supple skin. As a result, heavy drinkers also tend to wrinkle prematurely and, in general, age more quickly than others who consume alcohol sparingly or not at all.

Alcohol dehydrates, draining the skin of its plump, dewy appearance and directly damaging the Liver. Drinkers may appear sallow-complexioned and have dark circles under their eyes, as the Liver works harder to cleanse the body. Because they generally have more muscle than fat, men are able to digest alcohol more easily than women, so the ravages of drinking, either chronic or in occasional binges, take a heavier toll on women.

Smoking, 吸烟 *(xī yān)*

It is difficult to reconcile the "glamour" associated with smoking in movies and other media images with the ugly reality that smoking is another lifestyle choice that kills both inner and outer beauty.

In TCM, the Lung is intimately connected with the skin and the hair. When we think about the way in which the skin absorbs and emits substances, both nourishing and toxic, this makes sense: it is almost as if the skin is an external Lung, breathing from the outside of the body. Just as the internal Lung separates the inside from the outside, letting in the outside air and extracting nutrients from it, so does the skin.

When the Lung works normally, the skin and hair are nourished so that the skin has the density and the strength to repel external pathogens. If Lung Qi is deficient and weak, the skin and hair will lack nourishment and moisture: the skin will turn rough and dry, and the hair will look dull and weak. The interstices will loosen and make the skin vulnerable to disease.

If the diffusing function of the Lung is healthy, the skin's pores will regulate sweat correctly to meet the body's requirements. It is consistent, then, that smoking, which involves drawing heated fumes into the Lung, ends up affecting the skin. In TCM, that which weakens the Lung also affects the quality of the senses of taste and smell. This is certainly the case with smoking, as many studies have shown. The Lung is also associated with sadness, and I cannot help thinking that many heavy smokers appear to have lines expressing sadness in their faces, as opposed to the joyful lines created by a life of love and laughter.

It is widely known and accepted that smoking causes lung cancer and many other forms of cancer, heart failure, strokes, sexual impotence and birth defects, slow healing, shortened life-spans and greatly reduced quality of life. As with heavy drinkers, heavy smokers age prematurely, as their skin wrinkles and becomes sallow. This is because smoking accelerates the enzymes that break down collagen and elastin, which keep the skin dewy, moist and elastic, contributing to the acceleration of wrinkling.

Given this depressing litany of ills, I am pleased to see how much smoking has receded as an acceptable activity in North America. Even in diehard smoking societies such as France and Greece, it is becoming less respectable and increasingly illegal to smoke in public buildings. In this one area, China is still lagging, but I am hopeful that along with its lightning-fast modernization, the deadly habit will soon be the target of health reforms.

Smoking is a cause or a factor in such a long list of diseases and side effects that prevent the body from being balanced and healthy that I cannot think of a single greater contribution to your health and inner beauty than avoiding it. If you have never smoked, or have successfully quit, congratulations and keep it up!

Weight Gain, 体重增加 *(tǐ zhòng zēng jiā)*
There are many reasons why people gain weight. Sometimes it happens because they have tumours or other abnormal growths in their bodies—a situation that needs immediate medical

attention. Others gain weight because they expand their muscle mass through strenuous exercise. As long as they do not overdo it, this is usually a positive development for their overall health. But mostly, weight gain is the result of eating too much of the wrong kind of food, and not doing enough exercise.

Some people have a love affair with what they consume—or maybe it is just the idea of the food. They cannot resist shoving the food into their mouths as fast as they can—before they even taste it, and long before their poor overloaded brains can send the signal that enough is enough.

Sustainable weight loss is among the most challenging health issues that my patients and I confront. Even the most intelligent, rational people cannot seem to help gaining weight or, even worse, riding a roller coaster where their weight fluctuates wildly. They all understand how dangerous this is to their health and well-being, and yet they continue to do it. Why is this?

When I first came to Canada from China, I immediately concluded that either I had just arrived in a very rich country or there was a massive hormone imbalance in the general populace. So many overweight people! It took a while before I realized how widespread the problem was, and that many of my patients were at increased risk of diabetes, heart disease, cancer, stroke, sleep apnea and a host of other ailments. Many of my overweight patients are sad or alone. They suffer both physically and mentally.

It is easy to say that these patients eat too much and do not exercise enough. But the problem is far more complicated than that. Drive down any commercial street in North America, and you will be surrounded by opportunities to eat large servings of inexpensive fast food that is loaded with fat, salt, sugar and addictive chemicals. These foods are constantly advertised on large-screen televisions. In front of those screens are people who spend hours watching them without getting up to move around from time to time, or to prepare meals with fresh ingre-dients. Fast food is easy; preparing fresh and healthy food can be labour-intensive. It requires thinking constantly about what we are putting into our mouths. Many people do not know how to begin doing things differently.

TCM is concerned with the Toxins that patients carry in the extra layers of fat when they gain weight. It is no coinci-dence that people often gain weight when they are emotion-ally or chemically imbalanced. We support patients in returning to a healthy weight by detoxifying the Liver, supporting the Spleen's digestive function and helping the Kidney to stop retaining water.

In addition to TCM treatments, I find that many of my patients need advice about how to manage their own day-to-day routine. Sherry is a warm, wonderful woman who is universally admired by her colleagues and the many young people she has mentored over the years.

See page 204 for a herbal recipe to help with Liver detoxification and weight loss.

Her problem is that as she has risen in the ranks of her organization, the number of people who feel they need to talk to her every day has grown to the point that it is physically impossible for her to respond to the hundreds of emails and dozens of telephone calls that pour into her office every day—and that doesn't include the demands of her boss, who shows up at her door every few minutes because he values her advice so much.

One day, when someone asked Sherry how she had enjoyed the delicious homemade soup that she had eaten an hour earlier, she responded, "What soup?" She had no idea what the person was talking about. Since this colleague had gone to the trouble of making the soup at home and bringing it into the office espe-cially for her, Sherry was embarrassed, to say the least. Looking down at the dirty bowl on her desk, she realized that she had "inhaled" the soup so quickly, and so absent-mindedly, that she had no memory at all of its taste or even of approximately when she had eaten it. This voracious kind of eating leads directly to unhealthy weight gain.

It is not unusual for women, and even men, whose hormones slow down weight gain compared to women, to acquire fat layers that correspond to every promotion in the workplace—almost like morbid tree rings, year after year. As they become busier and more stressed, their own health and well-being often fall by the wayside.

I have been through several cycles with Sherry. Despite her position of power and her prominence, she is humble. She always agrees to follow my advice. For the first little while, she will eat with the seasons, do a fruit and vegetable cleanse, close her office door at lunchtime and chew her food slowly without multi-tasking. Inevitably, as she travels on business, as the work-load expands and her backlog of messages piles up, Sherry forgets my advice and returns to her old habits.

She knows that unless she promotes the new good habits to the level of her ongoing consciousness, nothing will truly change. I worry that the cycles of weight gain and loss will have long-term bad consequences for her health, but I cannot carry the whole load in helping her. And frankly, none of us is perfect when it comes to eating habits. Even I sometimes read while eating absent-mindedly. It is a constant effort to maintain a healthy lifestyle.

For some patients, carrying extra weight can be a form of protective armour against stress or a hostile world. Geraldine is an energetic, vigorous woman who had two babies while running a busy hypnotherapy practice. She was carrying significant excess weight. When I checked her pulse and her tongue, it was obvious to me that she had a Kidney Yang Deficiency.

But she could not believe it: "No way! I get more done in an hour than anybody!"

I told Geraldine that her strong mind had been keeping her going but that her body was too tired to follow. This is why she was using food to bolster her energy and her spirits. She was able to keep going this way, but only at the expense of weight gain and mood swings.

I put her on a detox program that included infrared saunas with herbal detoxing footbaths, and weekly acupuncture and herbs to increase her Kidney Yang. Geraldine says that her TCM treatments also helped her mentally and spiritually: "I finally got real and stopped pretending, started being authentic and honest. And I physically, completely, 100 per cent changed. My body has shed forty pounds, even though I work out less than ever. I've gone to a different place."

Geraldine began to understand that her body was dealing with a constant barrage of toxicity because she was living in opposition to her own true self. She said, "When you use the energy to transform and stop resisting—I stopped needing so much physical space, physical build. I opened right up. People who have seen me through it say that I look physically different: my skin is softer, and everything about me has changed."

Before this transformation, Geraldine would never have appeared anywhere without full makeup. Now she is comfortable with her natural, open, fresh face, and she actually appears to have shed years with the pounds. Geraldine's reflections on her own transformation have led her to believe that women do not exercise one important power that they have: the power not to purchase products that prey on their fears about their own beauty. "You don't need makeup, makeup needs you," she said. "The beauty shines through anyone when they are honest about what and who they are. It doesn't matter what you look like or physically how you are represented, but when you land on the truth of who you are, and you deliver this to the world by virtue of sharing it, or speaking it, or whatever that delivery is, you actually physically change."

Geraldine's success seems stable, but for some patients the challenges are continual.

Lifestyles can also change dramatically as a result of trauma, which can precipitate a series of domino effects that have far-reaching consequences for a person. It is very challenging to bring back such patients to consistent good health. Most often, lifestyle changes are crucial to the success of these efforts.

When I first met Penelope, she was in constant pain as a result of a debilitating injury that had significantly impaired her mobility. In the immediate aftermath of her injury, she had been encouraged to consume large amounts of non-steroidal anti-inflammatory drugs, and she had not been careful enough to always take them with food. As a result, she had developed serious stomach lesions and decided to stop taking the drugs.

This left Penelope with the challenge of keeping up an extremely demanding and high-pressure workload all day while ignoring her constant pain. The pain also discouraged her from exercising and caused her a great deal of stress. At the end of her long workdays, to comfort herself and to take her mind off the pain, she would eat too much of the food she enjoyed and drink a few glasses of wine. As she explained to me, "Wine is my painkilling drug of choice. I love it, I know how it affects me and I know when I have had enough."

Even if that were true, the problem was that wine contains a lot of calories, in addition to the food that was not proportionate to her sedentary work life. Over time, her weight crept up and added to the stress on her joints, her mobility issues and her pain. To compound her troubles, Penelope was entering early menopause and suffering from hot flashes and mood swings.

I was able to relieve Penelope's menopause symptoms easily and quickly with herbs and acupuncture, and she was very relieved to find that she was sailing relatively benignly through her Second Spring—something she had feared. Her TCM treatments also helped with pain management. But the weight issue was a stubborn one and seemed to be related to ongoing stress from work issues in her life.

After a few years, the work issues eased, and Penelope made up her mind to lose the weight. She went to a clinic that promoted a drastic weight loss method. I supported her with acupuncture and herbs to maintain her energy levels as she lost fifty pounds in five months, but I was worried about her. In my experience, quick and easy methods rarely yield lasting results.

Sure enough, gradually over the next two years, the stress returned to Penelope's life, and her weight went back up with it. She came to me and said, "Xiaolan, this time I'd like to do it your way. What do you think I should do?"

Since it was spring, I suggested it was the perfect time to do a juice fast using vegetables, including dark leafy greens, to return her body to an alkaline state. I told her she should prepare at least three litres a day of thick, healthy vegetable juices in a cold-press juicer to preserve the precious enzymes that would help relieve her congested body. I also suggested that she drink alkaline water as much as possible.

See page 181 for recipes for herbal remedies to deal with weight loss and stretch marks.

Penelope has not yet begun to follow this advice, as she is currently travelling a great deal and cannot have access to the fresh juice on a regular basis. She has agreed that she will schedule a three-week vegetable juice fast when she is able, followed by long-term changes in her diet.

I continue to be concerned about Penelope. However, knowing her determination when she puts her mind to something,

I am confident that with my support, she will succeed in losing the excess weight and sustaining her improved health. I also know another thing: along with the weight, many of her other health issues, such as digestive problems and arthritic change—will also subside. This will eliminate some problems and reduce others, making a major contribution to restoring her quality of life.

Clearly, in Penelope's case, stress played a role in weight gain, but there were also other determining factors, including those resulting from her original injury. One of the reasons I worry about her is that these factors, along with lifestyle issues, are increasing her risk of breast cancer, which has become a virtual epidemic in Western society. One in four of my female patients has developed it—a higher rate than in the general population in Canada, which is one in nine.

My patient Cally developed the disease at the young age of thirty-eight. She had been under great stress from a demanding job in her family business, and she was carrying a significant burden of excess weight. She wasn't eating properly and did not exercise. She kept herself going with six to eight cups of coffee a day. Self-conscious about her weight, Cally would starve herself during the day, only to find herself ravenous by late evening, when she would give in to her cravings and eat a large dinner just before going to bed.

When, after six years of marriage, she did not become pregnant on demand, she turned to an in vitro fertilization (IVF) clinic, where she was pumped full of hormones. When she developed breast cancer instead of getting pregnant, she was deeply shocked. Not only was her body not listening to her, it was betraying her.

Cally's feelings of "why me?" were not unusual. Most people who develop serious illnesses ask the same question. I asked her to look back at her lifestyle. To me, the warning signs were all there. Not unusual among North American women, Cally felt that she had no room in her life to do things solely for her own health and well-being. When I asked her why she lived like this, she could not answer. She had no real connection with her body.

To her credit, Cally reacted intelligently and diligently. From the moment that she came to us for help, she took serious steps to change her lifestyle and recover her health.

Her cancer had indeterminate borders, so her Western doctors recommended chemotherapy first. This was followed by a double mastectomy, radiation and a five-year course of tamoxifen. Throughout this process, and supported by her loving husband, she made dramatic changes in her life. First, she quit her job. She began juicing organic vegetables, eating several servings of organic fruit every day, and drinking lots of water. She began to understand that her body needed respect and tender loving care: she learned to massage her large areas of scar tissue twice a day using herbal oils. Gradually, she lost weight—an important step, since Toxins tend to be stored in adipose tissues. The colour began to return to her face, and her eyes began to shine. Ironically, she was much happier than she had been before her breast cancer.

For a description of breast cancer and its consequences, as well as recipes for herbal remedies, see page 95.

Cally came to us for regular treatments, including acupuncture, infrared saunas and Chinese herbs. She set out on a spiritual path to find inner peace, and began meditating and practising yoga. She is truly transformed, and radiates with inner beauty.

While I am not suggesting that IVF treatments cause breast cancer, I am concerned that the hormones used to stimulate fertility are among the kinds of interventions that shock the body and disturb its balance. In Cally's case, her body was already signalling an imbalance through her inability to conceive, her excess weight and her stress levels. The last time she saw her Western oncologist, he told her that he was very happy with her results: "Whatever you're doing, keep it up!"

YOU ARE WHAT YOU EAT

According to Western medicine, humans digest and assimilate food through their digestive system, which it defines more narrowly than the TCM view of a whole body system comprised of five Organ systems: Liver, Heart, Spleen, Lung and Kidney. TCM dietary recommendations take into account this added complexity.

Since the human body is 70 per cent water by weight, it makes sense that hydration is extremely important. TCM also emphasizes the pH of water, and the importance of alkaline water in preventing and treating cancer, which thrives in an acidic terrain.

Diet is an important element in a gentle self-care regimen, which also includes taking care of our emotional health and undertaking moderate physical activity. TCM makes specific dietary recommendations according to the time of life and the person's condition. In general, cold foods and fluids and raw and frozen foods are believed to be difficult for the Spleen and the Stomach to digest—even perhaps injuring the Qi. The effect of this is to slow the transformation process of food into Essence, or Jing, slow down the work of the Spleen and lead to Spleen Qi Deficiency, which hinders the overall flow of Qi in the body.

As with everything in TCM, diet is also a matter of balance. For example, overeating at one sitting overwhelms the Spleen and taxes its ability to extract Food-Qi, weakening the Spleen over time. Not eating enough, or eating irregularly, does not allow the Spleen to produce enough Food-Qi, and leads eventually to Deficient Qi and Blood.

Heavenly Water

The Liver and Kidney Organ systems govern a healthy flow of Heavenly Water, and trouble with menses generally starts from there. It is important to ensure that these systems are working well. Excessive consumption of cold foods and fluids, raw foods and frozen foods, over time, can create accumulations of Cold and Dampness, produce pain in the joints and increase bloating, cramping and discomfort during the time of Heavenly Water. The Spleen's proper functioning is very important to menstruation, since it ensures that Blood stays within the vessels and does not seep into the tissues. A Spleen Qi Deficiency can trigger a Blood Deficiency, insomnia or skipped menstrual periods, heavy menstrual flow, cramps with cold hands and feet, diarrhea and digestive problems.

Even slightly cooked foods are easier to digest than raw ones, and their nutrients are more readily absorbed. Hot drinks and soups can help to alleviate menstrual pain. However, coffee, alcohol, hot and spicy foods and large servings of red meat can stagnate the free movement of Liver Qi during Heavenly Water.

For my mother's egg soup and sweet rice congee recipes to alleviate menstrual pain, see page 136.

Rich, fatty or fried foods, excessive dairy products and raw foods will affect the free movement of both Liver and Spleen Qi and can cause a Spleen Qi Deficiency, Qi Stagnation and Dampness, depression and loss of energy.

One theory in TCM is that the Liver is an assertive, sometimes even aggressive Organ system, while the Spleen needs support. If the Liver becomes engorged with Qi because of stress and emotional disturbances prior to the onset of menses, this weakens the Spleen and triggers cravings for sweet foods. During Heavenly Water, such cravings—not only for sweet foods but also for chocolate and coffee—can deepen the level of Stagnation and Spleen Deficiency.

The caffeine in chocolate and coffee may temporarily move stagnant Qi, but it ends up causing a rebound effect. A high-fat diet also increases Qi Stagnation and Dampness, increasing the chances of low energy and depression. Reducing the intake of dairy foods and raw foods will, correspondingly, reduce Dampness and avoid taxing the Spleen.

Excess salt can also create a Kidney Deficiency that may result in water retention, lower back pain or urinary tract infections. Dark green leafy vegetables such as spinach, kale and dandelion leaves, red meat, liver, poultry, sweet rice, fish, eggs and raisins are all beneficial in replenishing Blood lost during Heavenly Water.

During the flow of Heavenly Water, take special care of yourself: maintain a regular and balanced schedule for eating, sleeping, working, exercising and resting. Avoid strenuous exercise and emotional stress.

Lotus Blossoms

A diet that promotes the free flow of Liver Qi is also the best way to promote the health of our breasts. Since Qi is warm, any time that it slows down, it can produce damaging Heat. Hot, spicy, peppery or fatty foods, too much red meat or alcohol, chocolate and caffeine are stimulants and produce Heat. They should be consumed in moderation. Foods that excite Qi disturb the balance that must be maintained between Qi and Blood throughout the system by drawing Qi to the surface of the body.

The foods that lead to Spleen Qi Stagnation—cold, frozen, raw and greasy foods, and dairy products—also tend to lead to the formation of Dampness, which damages the Spleen's ability to transform and transport fluids. This may result in the formation of Phlegm, one of the key contributors to the development of breast masses.

A well-balanced diet with a variety of foods, eaten in moderate amounts and regularly, is an excellent way to support breast health. These recommendations become even more important to support the body after treatment for breast cancer.

Ripening the Fruit

Many women suffer from morning sickness or nausea during pregnancy. This is because their Stomach Qi is blocked and is moving upward instead of downward. This may be caused by eating cold, raw and frozen foods, drinking cold fluids, worrying too much or overworking, or by physical or emotional exhaustion. Any of these factors can cause an imbalance in the Meridians that influence the flow of Stomach Qi. Balancing this flow is very important to Ripening the Fruit.

During pregnancy, it is important to drink lots of fluid and to avoid processed foods. Ginger is very helpful in treating nausea. We can make tea with fresh ginger, mint and honey or with fresh ginger and orange peel, and ginger rice (see recipes on pages 149 to 150).

When we are Ripening the Fruit, our diet should support the baby's growth and development. When I was pregnant with my son, Zhao Zhao, I ate many kinds of nuts and seeds, especially walnuts, almonds and sesame seeds, which contain essential fats for brain development. Walnuts even look like brains or Kidneys, and they are thought to increase Kidney Qi. I ate more fish, which also contains beneficial oils for brain development.

Since I wanted to make sure that my baby's bones and teeth were strong, I ate gallons of soup made from vast quantities of beef, pork and chicken bones. Adding two tablespoons of apple cider vinegar to the soup helps extract the calcium from the bones. In China, milk, whether soy or dairy, is not considered a good source of calcium, since it is believed to lead to the formation of Dampness that can impede the smooth flow of Qi.

During childbirth, a woman uses up Yang energy to push the baby out of the uterus, and loses a great deal of Blood. After childbirth, many small meals a day will strengthen Spleen Qi and replenish Kidney Essence without overtaxing the Spleen system. To regain the lost Yang, or Heat, the mother should eat Yang foods that are warming, such as lamb and other red meats, red kidney beans and lentils. My mother's egg soup (see recipe on page 136) helps to build Spleen Qi and enrich Blood.

Hair loss and postpartum depression are directly related to Blood loss. A new mother who has insufficient Blood in the Heart will feel lethargic, unable to sleep or bond with her baby, depressed, sad and anxious. This makes sense if we think that the spirit, or Shen, resides in the Heart.

It is important for the new mother to eat foods that nourish the Blood and support the Heart, Kidneys, Liver and Spleen, such as chicken, fish, green leafy vegetables, eggs, raisins, sweet rice and dried longan fruit. Eating chicken soup—almost universally recognized for its medicinal virtues—is an excellent way to replenish fluids, increase Yang energy, nourish Blood and dispel the Cold state of the body. The addition of motherwort herb (*Herba leonuri,* 益母草, yì mǔ cǎo) to the soup helps the Uterus regain its normal size and tone, and prevents excessive bleeding related to a Deficiency in the uterus.

Breastfeeding

Breastfeeding mothers need lots of fluids to sustain their milk flow, which requires both adequate Blood and Qi. They should avoid spicy, overly rich and greasy dishes, and foods that are not easily digested, such as raw foods and legumes. Bone soups, which contain marrow, will help to nourish Blood, Essence and the Kidneys, and may also help to prevent the joint pain that many women experience after childbirth. In China, the most traditional food for promoting lactation is pork hock boiled in black vinegar and ginger, as well as papaya and peanuts.

Second Spring

As we move out of our reproductive years and into Second Spring, we are living on our stored Kidney Qi and experiencing the consequences of choices we have made throughout our lives. Anything that supports the Kidneys and facilitates the free movement of Qi will help to prevent unnecessary erosion or consumption of our postnatal Essence and bring Yin and Yang back into balance.

We can do this proactively through diet by eating nutritious and balanced meals at regular intervals. Eating after eight o'clock in the evening creates a burden for the Spleen by leaving food in the Stomach overnight. This means the Spleen needs to work harder, or draw on the Kidney for additional Qi, or Heat, to transform and transport the food. The body will also have to produce more Heat to counterbalance the Cold, leading to less moisture and more hot flashes, as well as weight gain.

As Qi flows through the Stomach and Spleen systems between seven and eleven in the morning, it is important to have a warm, nutritious breakfast of foods that are agreeable to these Organs. The following chart is a good guide to the recommended diet for Second Spring.

It is important throughout life to be physically active. In Second Spring and old age, gentler forms of exercise such as Tai Chi and Qi Gong are highly recommended. My parents started taking Tai Chi classes when they were forty and have practised it every day since. It keeps them supple and healthy, and my mother has completely overcome her old knee problem.

Lifelong health and inner beauty depend heavily on nutrition and lifestyle—and common sense, which is not nearly as common as we would like it to be.

TABLE 2: DIETARY RECOMMENDATIONS FOR SECOND SPRING

AVOID OR REDUCE	GOOD CHOICES
• Cold foods and drinks • Frozen foods • Raw foods • Dairy products • Rich, fatty foods • Greasy foods • Sugar and refined carbohydrates • Coffee • Alcohol • Carbonated soft drinks • Hot and spicy foods • Large amounts of red meat	• Cooked foods, served warm • Lightly cooked fresh vegetables • Dark green leafy vegetables, dried longan fruit, liver, eggs, raisins • Almonds, walnuts, sunflower seeds, pumpkin seeds • Bone soups • Soy products • String beans, kidney beans, black beans • Mung beans and sprouts • Black sesame seeds • Seaweed • Oily fish such as sardines, salmon, tuna, mackerel • Whole grains

Cancer

So many of my patients have cancer that I am forced to think about this family of diseases every day. Understanding the potential of food as medicine is crucial in preventing and fighting cancer. This is an area where Western medicine and TCM differ greatly in their emphasis on treatment versus healing, but together they can be very complementary.

· The Western approach is to treat cancer by killing the cancerous cells with chemotherapy or radiation, or removing them surgically whenever possible. The TCM approach is to work with the body's unyielding capacity to heal itself. This includes helping patients deal with their emotions and mindset and their nutrition, as well as balancing their energy to achieve homeostasis, a condition in which the body is able to combat disruptions to maintain its equilibrium. It is possible to experience healing without successful treatment of the cancer.

Physicians and patients struggle constantly with the vast range of different kinds of cancer cells that can invade healthy tissues. It is truly the epidemic of our time. Despite their versatility, however, these cancers all have one thing in common that holds some hope for patients: all cancer cells need oxygen and energy, which come from blood vessels. Tumours are constantly finding ways to stimulate the growth of new blood vessels (angiogenesis, from the Greek words *angio,* meaning "vessel," and *genesis,* meaning "creation") to feed their abnormal growth and to invade surrounding tissues.

One of the most promising ways to prevent and treat cancer is to find ways to block or destroy these new and specialized blood vessels, whose only purpose is to feed tumours. In the pharmaceutical field, antiangiogenic drugs that do this are sometimes called "metronome" therapies, because they tick away like the musician's tool rather than flooding the body in cycles, like the powerful cellular poisons contained in chemotherapy drugs. This makes them much more benign than chemotherapy, which can have devastating effects on the body as it kills rapidly multiplying healthy cells in mucous tissues and hair follicles along with the cancer cells.

The good news is that many fruits and vegetables contain some of these antiangiogenic molecules. Some foods are recommended because they inhibit angiogenesis, or because they are rich in the antioxidants and indole-3-carbinol that promote healthy cell growth and help to prevent cancer. These foods include green tea, cooked tomatoes, blueberries, prunes, raisins, garlic, dark leafy greens such as spinach and kale, and cruciferous vegetables high in indole-3-carbinol, such as broccoli, cauliflower, Brussels sprouts and cabbage, as well as red wine (in moderation, of course!). Many of these foods also contain two important antioxidants, lutein and zeaxanthin.

Foods rich in folate are important to the methylation process, which detoxifies harmful compounds from the body. This B vitamin is available in many foods, including orange juice, cereals, spinach, romaine lettuce, Brussels sprouts, asparagus, dried beans and peas. It is important to have adequate levels of folate because it has been shown to protect against the DNA mutations found in cancer processes.

Garlic contains allium compounds that support the immune system. Turmeric, a member of the ginger family, helps fight cancer by promoting digestion and healing the intestines. It also contains curcumin, which has been shown to be a powerful anti-inflammatory. Hot chili peppers, including jalapenos, contain capsaicin, which is widely believed to be a cancer-fighting agent.

Oranges and lemons stimulate the immune system to reduce cancer cells, and also contain the antioxidant vitamin C. This miracle vitamin can be found in many fruits and vegetables, including papayas and raspberries, which also contain many other vitamins and minerals that help to protect against cancer. The ideal form of vitamin C is in whole foods such as broccoli, cabbage, Brussels sprouts, legume sprouts, parsley and sauerkraut.

Juicing raw fruits and vegetables allows the body to absorb their nutrients more immediately into the bloodstream, which is especially important in certain types of cancers and other illnesses where the digestive process is compromised. Juicing also preserves the precious living enzymes in these foods, which play an important role in optimizing the metabolic processes. Cooking, processing and oxidation, which results from leaving the foods or the juices around for too long before consuming them, kills their enzymes. Cofactors are the minerals and vitamins required to fuel the enzymatic reaction.

Vitamin D is another potent anti-cancer agent and has been shown to improve survival rates among lung cancer patients. The research suggests that the recommended daily dose of vitamin D should be increased to 1,000 IU for both men and women. Although vitamin D is usually associated with dairy products, high concentrations also can be found in eggs, cod, shrimp and chinook salmon. Ten minutes of sunshine on 40 per cent of your body without sunscreen can generate as much as 5,000 IU of vitamin D. People living in temperate climates where they expose little skin to the sun most of the year (such as in Canada, where I live) are most at risk of vitamin D deficiency.

The antioxidants in nuts may help to suppress the growth of tumours. One example is Brazil nuts, which contain the antioxidant selenium.

Calcium and magnesium (which is necessary for calcium's absorption) are also an important part of any cancer protocol, to protect bones and promote healthy sleep. Certain foods are calcium inhibitors and should be consumed carefully and in moderation, reduced or eliminated. These include coffee, soft drinks and diuretics, excesses of protein, especially meat, refined sugar or too much of any concentrated sweetener or sweet-flavoured food, alcohol, marijuana, cigarettes and other intoxicants and salt. Too little or too much exercise will also inhibit the absorption of calcium.

All teas are good for the body, although drinking too much black or green tea can be acidifying and drying. Tea contains antioxidant flavonoids; kaempferol is especially protective against cancer. Green tea has the highest concentration of polyphenol antioxidants.

THE SOY CONTROVERSY

In Asian countries soy is an important part of the general diet. It seems no coincidence that there are far fewer hormone-fed cancers such as breast cancer and prostate cancer in Asia than in North America and Europe, as well as much lower reporting of unpleasant symptoms during menopause. In addition, survival rates for breast cancer are higher among Asian women. There are many reasons why this might be so, including the rich iso-flavone content of soybeans and products derived from them. They also contain genistein, which is both a plant estrogen and an antiangiogenic molecule that helps to prevent the appearance of tumours. There may be an additional protective effect if these soy-based foods are consumed since before puberty.

It is best to consume whole soy foods such as raw edamame or dry-roasted soybeans (about 50 grams a day) to benefit from the anti-cancer effects of isoflavones. Supplements are not an acceptable alternative to these whole foods.

However, for some women, including those who develop breast tumours while their estrogen levels are low, isoflavones may trigger rapid growth of these tumours. This may happen because the compounds are similar in chemical structure to sex hormones. As a result, they may interfere with the development of cancers caused by high levels of these hormones in the body. I recommend that in these situations, you consult your physician or nutritionist before deciding whether to consume these foods, and in what amounts.

Every day, it is within your power to make the right choices to ensure that your body is balanced with the right foods, plenty of exercise and sleep. TCM recognizes the body's ability to heal itself: by listening closely to your body's signals and meeting its needs, you will be supporting your inner health and beauty.

CHAPTER SEVEN

SECOND SPRING AND GROWING OLD

第二春 *(dì èr chūn)*

Man fools himself. He prays for a long life and he fears old age.
—*Chinese proverb*

The emperor is rich, but he cannot buy one extra year.
—*Chinese proverb*

S econd Spring is an end and a beginning. It is the end of fertility and youth, the bodily experience of our impermanence. It is also the beginning of a new and vital stage of life—a time of liberation from responsibilities, when we are freed to reinvest our energies in ourselves, both physically and psychologically. Many women find that in Second Spring, they gain insight and understanding that empower them to feel more capable, more competent and more confident than ever before in their lives.

This is a time of life when women travel, start businesses and pick up new sports and hobbies. No longer responsible for young children, they enjoy their freedom to explore, to invent and to create. They become leaders and innovators.

After studying fine arts as a young girl, Laura concentrated on raising her three children and supporting her working husband for many years. She arranged her entire life around their needs and their happiness, setting aside her own ambitions and desires. When the children were grown up, she felt the deep satisfaction of knowing that they had all found fulfilling careers in the fields of their choice. With Second Spring, she recognized in herself a need to create: she returned to her roots in the arts and became a painter. She felt as if she had picked up where she had left off, the young woman with the fine arts degree growing into a respected artist with an international following.

Another patient, Lisa, worked very hard and raised four children alone after divorcing her husband. Once the children had left the house, she found that she had a new passion: children in Africa, who had so much less than her own children had enjoyed growing up. She used her new-found freedom to set up a school in Africa, finding deep happiness in making a difference in the lives of these little ones, very far from her original home. Seeing her commitment, her children supported her unconditionally in these choices. Lisa was reaping the fruits of her life as a devoted mother in her Second Spring of adventure and freedom.

Until they experience it for themselves, many of my patients do not see the wonderful side of Second Spring. As we work together to keep them healthy and balanced through this period of transition, then they are often surprised at something that TCM explains very well: the positive side of the end of fertility.

> Enjoy yourself. It's later than you think.
> —Chinese proverb

For all of their fertile years, women's bodies devote huge amounts of Qi to a Herculean task: every twenty-eight days or so, they set aside a portion of their nutrition, oxygen and stored resources to prepare a nutritious and welcoming environment, just in case a fertilized egg lands in the uterus. Every twenty-eight days, if no such egg lands, they give up these resources in the form of menstrual blood—only to start all over again. This happens every single month, from adolescence until Second Spring, except in the time during and right after pregnancy.

Until they experience it for themselves, women don't realize how physically and psychologically liberating Second Spring will be. Imagine being able to reinvest all of that energy into your own life, for your own purposes! This is a revelation for many women. When this energy is harnessed to wisdom, it makes women a formidable force in Second Spring. And this strength is necessary in so many ways.

> Yellow gold is plentiful compared to white-haired friends.
> —*Chinese proverb*

This is a time when our own parents become old and fragile, and our children may be having children of their own, needing our support. We begin to see serious illnesses and deaths among those our own age, forcing us to recognize our own impermanence and the brevity of our lives. All of these developments move us toward forgiveness and letting go of the things that do not truly matter. We are able to feel compassion for friends, our families and ourselves. We are open to the realm of Shen, the spiritual. In Second Spring, women gain the strength, the wisdom and the desire to connect with the deeply meaningful, and to let go of that which is not.

This is also a time when knowledge about managing our health becomes more important than ever. With declining Kidney Qi comes a need to think more carefully about food as medicine. Preserving Qi requires making sure we have the right kinds of food to concentrate, to function and to enjoy our lives.

In societies like the one in which I was raised in China, where the generations live together, there is a continuum of knowledge and wisdom that is always being transferred to new generations. Families congregate around birthing mothers and are closely involved in supporting the young family afterwards. Grandparents take care of their grandchildren and are closely involved in their lives. They are highly respected and treasured for this teaching. In turn, they derive great fulfillment from the feeling of nurturing and helping the younger generation to learn. In letting go of their own egos, living in the moment with younger people, they gain peace and serenity.

> The house with an old grandparent harbours a jewel.
> —*Chinese proverb*

I see examples of this wisdom among my patients. Heather is a ninety-one-year-old actress who lives every day in serenity and peace. She still works regularly, performing with enjoyment and gusto on stage and on screen—although she sometimes has to rely on her sense of humour, given the kinds of roles that are available for a woman of her age. She lives alone in a beautiful home, filled with her paintings and flowers from her garden. She writes poetry and letters to her children and grandchildren, and even a great-grandchild, whose lives she follows from afar. Because she is lively and wonderful company, they all enjoy their visits with her whenever they can.

Heather loves coming to my clinic every two weeks—not only because it helps her maintain her health and well-being, but because it represents an opportunity for her skin to be touched in a caring way. She lost her loving husband a number of years ago and misses the physical closeness and affection that she enjoyed with him over a long period of time. This is something that many older people need and do not receive often enough, particularly as their sexual lives diminish—often not by their choice.

Beautiful young people are accidents of nature, but beautiful old people are works of art.

—ELEANOR ROOSEVELT

We appreciate her visits for many reasons, not least because Heather's generous laugh resonates through our clinic and brings us joy. All of my colleagues enjoy giving her treatments, because there is something in her energy that makes us feel that whatever we give her comes back to us in a beautiful way.

On a wall in Heather's house is a triptych that she painted a few years ago. It is a simple pot of tulips, but she has captured their beauty in three stages: "I painted them week one, standing up and fresh, then I painted them week two when they were mature, and the petals were opening, and then I painted them week three, when the petals were the colour of this jacket [black], and they were still beautiful." Heather is right. Her passion for life and beauty in all its forms is inspiring. She understands that for all living beings, our time is over quickly. Somehow she has found the wisdom to live consciously in the present moment, and the confidence to know that she is beautiful. Whatever she is doing, she never forgets to be.

My patient Deanna, at fifty, radiates with health and beauty. She has enjoyed a close relationship with her elderly relatives, and great insight into the value and beauty of their lives. Recently, she talked to me about the death of her ninety-four-year-old mother-in-law, a beloved patient who came to our clinic every three weeks for many years: "She got more and more beautiful as she aged, with a unique style about her. There was a certain peacefulness—when that woman got out of her life, she didn't have to be anything to anybody. She loved coming here, because [otherwise] she never was touched. It starts with children being touched and goes all the way to the elderly.

For TCM treatments of skin conditions in old age, see page 206.

If you don't have anybody left in your life and there's nobody touching you, it's just something that you miss. Personal contact is so important. So I think that really enhanced her life and extended it, coming to see Xiaolan. She did love you, and she loved to come and talk to you. But she'd be so happy to get her feet rubbed, her hands. She would come back and her cheeks would be pink."

How did I grow to come from a poor, poor house and a poor family and to be able to find all this beauty in the world and to hold it in my hands? To learn how to grow gorgeous flowers, those roses out there, the beans that I grew this summer, the runty little tomatoes this year, the great herbs—I see beauty everywhere: in skin, in hair, in the petals of flowers, in earth, the colour of the soil, the colour of wood.

—HEATHER, NINETY-ONE-YEAR-OLD PATIENT

CONCLUSION

You have to do your own work;
those who have reached the goal will only show the way.

If the roots remain untouched and firm in the ground,
a felled tree still puts forth new shoots.
If the underlying habit of craving and aversion is not
uprooted, suffering arises anew over and over again.

—*the Buddha,* Dhamapada

My clinic is a bustling little town. Over the course of a year, more than twelve thousand patients come through our doors. Each one of them rightly expects that each one of us on staff will focus entirely on them when they are with us. We therefore need to be strong, focused and resilient if we are to preserve the personal essence that this work requires.

For many years, since I finished medical school at the age of twenty-four, the most powerful tool I have found to support my work and my career has been daily meditation. It helps me with alertness, mental clarity, focus and much more. It has sustained me through years of change and hard work, and I would have to give it credit for much of my career success. This success, real as it is, has been achieved by the mind.

From the time we are born and open our eyes to see a mother, a father and all that life has to offer a curious little baby, very few of us ever turn our gaze inside ourselves. We know surprisingly little about ourselves. We are frequently alienated from our own bodies and consciousness. To complicate things further, we experience traumas throughout our lives that leave their mark on our bodies. These traumas continue to resonate through our bodies and our minds whenever we try to live in peace and serenity, from moment to moment.

Slowly, over the years, it has dawned on me that something has been missing. Since my late thirties, I have found increasing solace in Buddhism, my grandmother's tradition. Meditation has become a crucial part of my life, a daily way to centre myself in the here and now, and to gather strength.

I have learned a great deal from listening to others; I have succeeded in processing knowledge through intellectual analysis. I thought that I could always distinguish whether a patient was talking to me from the head or from the heart. But just as the eye cannot see itself, I did not understand that I, too, was operating almost entirely from the mental level.

It is hard to believe that something as small as a mosquito can cause an existential crisis, but that is exactly what happened to me. Mosquitoes are the one thing I cannot control with the force of my mind. No meditation technique will fix this. I know that if I am bitten I should not scratch—but I cannot help it! I need to scratch! And when I am bitten, I scratch the bites until they are bloody. Friends have put socks over my hands and arms to stop me, but this one thing is beyond my capacity to control. This may sound very strange, but facing this squarely tipped me over the edge: I needed to go much further to understand my own consciousness.

What I realized is that much as I valued my practice of meditation, it was not enough to help me accept the rising and passing of the atoms that make up my material being and the impermanence of everything around me with equanimity—not to mention mosquito bites! Without a tool to work through my direct experience of life, I could not truly achieve this deep understanding of how to live. I needed something more.

As I was finishing work on this book, I decided to give myself a gift: I would pursue a ten-day course at a Vipassana meditation retreat. Vipassana is a 2,500-year-old non-sectarian technique that helps us to see life as it really is. The entry to Vipassana is only through this ten-day course, which is available to anyone who wants to do it.

Vipassana teaches the art of living and being, and provides a universal remedy for human suffering. It helps us to transform ourselves through self-observation and to achieve a balanced mind, full of love and compassion, by focusing on the deep interconnection between mind and body. However, we can only do this through a focused and disciplined effort over a long period of time.

On arrival at the retreat, I relinquished all the things that identify me: my wallet, my BlackBerry, my car keys. However, I kept my medical bag full of acupuncture needles and herbs. It is always with me when I travel, in case someone needs my help. Being a physician is an important part of my identity—not only a physician, but a supremely healthy, physically strong one.

I knew that the first three days of the ten were about the basics of meditation. As a decades-long practitioner, I was very confident that I would sail through these introductory days. I was in for a few surprises!

The first surprise was at the dawn of the first day. As a life-long A student and a physician obsessed with excellence, I normally trust myself to execute any given task well. I had not even set my alarm, convinced that my healthy body would jump out of bed and respond to the gongs that summon the students to class and to meditation sessions. On the first morning, I woke happily until I realized that it was already 5:30—a full ninety minutes later than the official wake-up time!

Immediately, blood rushed to my head and triggered a

pounding headache. I felt flushed and hot. I was a failure already, on the first day! How could I have done this? How could I have slept in and missed the first gong? I reproached myself bitterly. I was angry at myself. I was ashamed to walk to the dining hall. I did not feel that I deserved to have the breakfast served by volunteers who get up before everyone else.

Intellectually, I understood that I was bone-tired after three years without a single true holiday. I had been so looking forward to this ten-day course—even though it would prove to be intense, hard work, and not the holiday that my body craved. But still, pride and a passion for excellence seem to be in my DNA. I could not control my body's reaction. It took me an hour to calm down. To my chagrin, there was a distinct gap between my intellectual capacity to let go and my body's refusal to follow orders from my mind.

I ate my breakfast in the prescribed noble silence of body, mind and voice. For the entire ten-day period, the hundred people in the course would neither read nor write, nor speak, nor even make eye contact. An hour-long breakfast under these conditions was a revelation—and very different from my usual grab-and-dash daily routine. Without any other distractions, I could actually taste and experience every bite of food. The sweetness, the textures, the goodness of the oats, the fruits, the herbal tea, the sensation of sesame seeds in my teeth—the intense awareness transformed the act of eating.

Once in the group meditation hall, we listened carefully to five minutes of taped instructions. The tape told us to observe the natural phenomenon of the rising and passing of our bodily sensations—whether they be pleasant or unpleasant—and to learn by experience of their impermanence. If the sensation was pleasurable, we were told not to attach ourselves to it. If it was unpleasant, we were to try not to develop strong emotions about it. No cravings; no aversions.

The first exercise was to remain completely still for two and a half hours and to focus exclusively on breathing in the small triangle formed by the nostrils and lips, observing and not judging "what is." As per the instructions, I placed my body in the position I believed would be most comfortable for me—the lotus position I use to meditate every day of my life. Again, I was certain this would be a piece of cake. My left knee had a different idea. In the silence and immobility, it began to speak up.

As my knee forced me to tune in to its frequency, it began to express itself. I tried to ignore it and remain focused only on my breathing, but my inner physician was instantly alert. My mind butted in and began to ask sharp questions. Where is this pain coming from? What happened to this knee? Why is it flaring now? Where should I be putting in needles to fix it? Again, my busy mind swooped in to diagnose and treat; I was proud of myself for having brought my bag. As soon as I could, I would do what I always do: I would treat myself before this painful knee could become a real problem.

Of course, the imperative was to remain completely still, but I could not help surreptitiously moving ever so slightly to try and shut down the yelping knee. Things just got worse. After an hour, the knee became emboldened by my obligation to observe and not react to bodily sensations. As I observed the pain, the knee spoke up louder and louder until it was screaming—so loudly that I could not even hear myself breathing. The pain was excruciating. Tears began to roll down my cheeks. Still I did not move—and slowly, my knee began to calm down. By the evening session, it was almost as if it had never happened.

I was not going to get off so easily, however. The next day, as I meditated again, a new pain crept up on me, from between my shoulder blades. Again, the pain grew until it was excruciating. It was so intense that I hallucinated—as if I had been stabbed in the back in another life. Unlike the previous day, this time I knew I could not treat myself. My busybody mind again butted in. It was already making mental appointments with the chiropractor and the craniosacral therapist; I was already assigning a member of my staff to give me acupuncture.

I was amazed: could this be my body? Was it possible that with all my training, I had been unaware of such acute latent problems in my own body? For the first time, I began to experience my patients' pain through the reality of my own senses. I felt myself moving from the intellectual understanding and compassion of a trained physician to the consciousness of a human being whose compassion is based on shared suffering.

I have attended births and deaths and almost every human experience in between, and I thought I knew how to handle these situations very well. What I had not realized was how deeply and universally we all share this passage through life and this suffering. And yet, we spend much of our lives separating ourselves from this inevitable suffering by refusing to accept the reality of it, and seeking to escape it.

We do this in many ways—through drugs, alcohol, sex, shopping, golf or work—whatever it takes for each one of us. None of these things works to actually stop the suffering, nor do they even stop our bodies from continuing to experience physiological reactions to these stresses. These diversions only trap us in a process of endless and accelerated craving for more that removes us from our own humanity and blinds us to the suffering of others.

Facing reality—truly facing it and accepting it—liberates us from this endless cycle of craving that is tied to our egos, our status, our position in society and our professional identities, and opens us up to the peace of the deeper human truth beyond it.

As I moved through the ten-day experience, the pain travelled through my body, ebbing and flowing. In my inner conversation, I said, "I have had lots of pain now. Please may I have some kind of pleasure—any kind of pleasure?"

On the eighth day, my wish was granted. The pain stopped completely. I felt light and clear. I was beyond pleasure. I had crossed the line from form to formlessness. I felt profoundly alive—as if I had finally, for the first time, found my inner purpose, what I had been looking for all my life. In these ten days, I lived—truly lived—my entire life.

I felt that I was the most fortunate person in the world to have this opportunity, this time and this teaching, with the support of my staff, my family, my friends and my old dog, Nangua, who co-operated by not encountering any major health problems for the entire time I was away.

In many ways, I did not find it easy to stop and do nothing but listen to my own body. For one thing, my thirty years of training to listen to other people's health needs made it very difficult to sit and concentrate on my own breathing while others around me were coughing and sneezing and cracking their bones. I was constantly reacting to these signals, worried that one person might be developing pneumonia, that another might be spreading the flu among our group, and that a third was developing a joint problem. The teachers protected me from the efforts of others to contact me about people's health issues. And amazingly, the world managed the ten days without me.

Why am I sharing this experience with you?

We all know that constant change is the inescapable reality. We are all born, we live, we love, we suffer and we die. And yet, knowing it intellectually is not enough. We must find a way to live our lives meaningfully despite constant change and despite the suffering of pain, illness, loss, aging and our own mortality. This means liberating ourselves from the suffering itself but also from the need to escape the suffering.

> He hath lived ill that knows not how to die well.
> —Chinese proverb

All of the world's religions and moral codes have in common the need for moral behaviour. They also have in common various ways and techniques to master our emotions and cravings. From anger management courses to deep spiritual renewal, all of these techniques have something to offer. Counting to ten before speaking intemperately is a good idea. But pushing our reactions down into ourselves where they can fester and explode elsewhere is not a solution. It is only by observing and accepting that impermanence, loss and death are not personal, but simply and universally what is, that we can become whole beings, living in serenity and peace.

All of us, particularly women, live in a cruel world where people are judged first and foremost by their appearance. This exerts constant pressure and causes constant pain because people do not feel free to simply be who they are. But we all have a choice in how we live our lives.

Each of us has such a short time here on earth. Many of the planet's animals and trees live far longer than humans. In geological terms, we are here for a nanosecond in comparison to the rocks and the lands that surround us. Each of us has a choice about how to live our lives. There is a simple story that illustrates this very well.

A mother has three sons. She sends the first son to buy oil. On his way home, he trips and falls and loses half the oil. He arrives home crying and upset at his misfortune, complaining that he was only able to save half the oil.

The following week, the mother sends her second son to buy oil. He too trips on his way home, losing half the oil. When he reaches home, he tells his mother how thankful he is that he was able to save half the oil. He tells her how happy he is that he did not injure himself when he fell.

The third week, the mother sends her third son, who has the same experience. Not only is he happy that he saved half the oil, but he is also industrious: he tells his mother that he is going straight back to the market and will be able to earn the money to replace the lost oil before the end of the day.

We all know on an intellectual level that we would like to be positive, happy and productive. We know that the present moment is all we have. But the truth is that very few people succeed in living this way every day. Many people live in anxiety, anger, grief and depression—especially when they face their own suffering, aging and illness.

I cannot tell you exactly how to go about making the right choices for yourself. But I do hope that this book will help you recognize that honouring the needs of your body and spirit is one of the most important things you can do. In this book, my friend Sandy and I have sought to give you knowledge and techniques to take better care of yourself, and tools to understand and treat illnesses. We have sought to explain the crucial links between health and beauty.

May your inner beauty shine for yourself, and for the world around you.

ACKNOWLEDGEMENTS

I had such a beautiful experience with my first book, *Reflections of the Moon on Water,* that I was delighted to work once again with the team at Random House Canada, beginning with Anne Collins, my wonderfully supportive publisher. From the outset, Anne loved the idea that inner health and balance radiate to the outside in the form of beauty that is meaningful and lasting. She understood how important this idea is amid the constant pressures from the media and the outside world to conform to artificial and non-existent standards of beauty that none of us can ever achieve, and that can only lead to suffering.

Senior editor Pamela Murray has been a font of quiet competence and clever ideas, helping me ensure that this book came together smoothly. I struggled with the way to marry the storytelling and philosophical aspects of this book with the practical information that people have been demanding of me. Miraculously, Pamela found a way to structure the book that would work for readers, and I am so grateful for her constructive and skilful advice. Stacey Cameron, who also edited my first book, was just as conscientious and impeccable in her work on this one. My thanks also go to Sharon Klein, the energetic, talented, multi-tasking and hard-working publicist at Random House who has obtained so much media coverage for me and my work.

I am grateful as well for the talents of associate director of production Carla Kean, designer Terri Nimmo and typesetter

Erin Cooper, who contributed so much to the inner and outer beauty of this book.

I asked my friend and long-time patient Pauline Couture to write this book with me because I believed that she would bring her gift for writing to bear on a subject that she understands from profound experience. In the course of working together, I gave her a Chinese name: 神笔 (shén bǐ), or Magic Pen, because she was able to express so quickly what was in my mind and my heart—and to navigate effortlessly among English, Mandarin characters, Pinyin and Latin! We worked long and hard, laughed a great deal and ate too much, but we got it done. I also want to thank Pauline's husband, Ian Morrison, who put up patiently with our hours and hours of closeted work and brought endless pots of tea.

Dr. Sandy Skotnicki is my friend and patient, but first and foremost a highly respected colleague: a Western dermatologist who is also a scientist, an academic and a skilled clinician. Sandy and I explored many ways in which we could collaborate to improve outcomes for our patients, and we share the dream of linking Eastern and Western wisdom for patient wellness. I particularly want to thank Sandy for the amount of time she devoted to this project, given her very busy schedule.

David Bray, a highly respected TCM practitioner and expert in international publishing standards for TCM herbal recipes, was invaluable to us in verifying the accuracy of the information in this book. He is the very best at what he does. Any remaining errors in the book are mine alone.

I want to thank my friends who read the manuscript throughout the process and gave us very helpful feedback: Linda Haynes, Diane Bald, Gabriella Martinelli, Ludwig Max Fischer, Lorraine Segato, Naomi Duguid, Wende Cartwright, Howard Sagar, David Battistella, Carlos Hernandez, Hans Burgschmidt, Scott Remborg, Ian Saville, Victor De Lanessan, Christine Waque,

Karen Minden, Sandra Lax, Wendy Yiu, Gary Gray, Ann Marie Keating, and Jin Zhao.

I owe a great debt of gratitude to Dr. Christina Gordon and her beautiful and very patient baby daughter, Sage, as well as to Greggor Hagley, who provided the magnificent baby pictures to illustrate the baby massage techniques in this book.

I also want to thank my dear friends Anka and Tom Czudec for the author photograph that appears on the cover. Their patience and understanding of the process of working with such a reluctant subject is a gift I value so much.

I have dedicated this book to my devoted and highly competent staff at the Xiaolan Health Centre, whose contribution to the health and well-being of our patients is simply immeasurable. This includes Nelia DaSilva, assisted by Liang Tao and Shan Shen, and the medical staff: Vicky (Wei) Dong, Li Li, Libby (Xu Li Qin), Helen (Hui Rong Zhang), Denise Boutilier, Mariko (Qing Yang), Amanda (Luizhen Pan), Lindsay MacMillan, M.D., Karen Swirsky, M.D. Christina Gordon, N.D., David Denis, N.D., and Shawn Rashotte, RMT.

Thank you to all the patients who shared their stories of healing and their wisdom to help others learn through this book.

I am blessed with a large number of wonderful friends, colleagues and loved ones who supported me through the long process of writing this book. During this time, I was unavailable or late for parties, outings and birthday gatherings, and I thank them all for understanding. And finally, thank you to my always loving and supportive family: my parents, my brother and sisters and their spouses, and my beloved son, Zhao Zhao.

MAJOR TCM AND ACUPUNCTURE ASSOCIATIONS

If you are interested in finding a TCM practitioner in your area, contact one of the following organizations for a recommendation:

CANADA
The Chinese Medicine and Acupuncture Association of Canada
154 Wellington St
London, ON N6B 2K8
Tel: 519-642-1970
www.cmaac.ca

The Canadian Society of Chinese Medicine and Acupuncture
245 Fairview Mall Dr, Unit 402
Toronto, ON M2J 4T1
Tel: 416-597-6769
Fax: 416-597-9928
www.tcmcanada.org

The Canadian Association of Acupuncture & Traditional Chinese Medicine
3195 Sheppard Ave E, 2nd Floor
Scarborough, ON M1T 3K1
Tel: 416-493-8447
Toll-free: 1-888-299-9799
Fax: 416-493-9450
www.caatcm.com

ALBERTA
College and Association of Acupuncturists of Alberta
Health Professions and Telehealth Branch
Alberta Health and Wellness
10th Floor, Telus Plaza North Tower
10025 Jasper Ave
Edmonton AB T5J 2N3
Tel: 780-422-2733
Toll-free (within Alberta): 310-0000, then dial 780-422-2733
Fax: 780-415-1094
www.acupuncturealberta.ca

BRITISH COLUMBIA
College of Traditional Chinese Medicine Practitioners and
Acupuncturists of British Columbia
1664 West 8th Ave
Vancouver BC V6J 1V4
Tel: 604-738-7100
Fax: 604-738-7171
www.ctcma.bc.ca

Traditional Chinese Medicine Association of British Columbia
300-5900 No. 3 Rd
Richmond BC V6X 3P7
Tel: 604-278-6220
www.tcmabc.org

NEWFOUNDLAND AND LABRADOR
The Chinese Medicine and Acupuncture Association of
Newfoundland and Labrador
47 Leslie St
St. John's NL A1E 2V7
Tel: 709-738-0158
Fax: 709-722-5527
www.cmaanl.com

ONTARIO
Ontario Association of Acupuncture and Traditional Chinese
Medicine
370 B Dupont St
Toronto, ON M5R 1V9
Tel: 416-944-2265
www.oaatcm.com

The Professional Association of Traditional Chinese Medicine
304-3601 Victoria Park Ave
Toronto, ON M1W 3Y3
Tel: 647-505-1957
Fax: 1-866-384-3450
tcmassociation.com

PRINCE EDWARD ISLAND
Association of Registered Acupuncturists of Prince Edward Island
44 Grafton St
Charlottetown PE C1A 1K5
Tel: 902-628-1478
www.acupuncturepei.com

QUEBEC
Order of Acupuncturists of Quebec/Ordre des acupuncteurs du Québec
505, boul. René-Lévesque ouest
bureau 1106
Montréal QC H2Z 1Y7
Tel: 514-523-2882
Toll-free: 1-800-474-5914
Fax: 514-523-9669
www.ordredesacupuncteurs.qc.ca

INTERNATIONAL
The Accreditation Commission for Acupuncture and Oriental Medicine
Maryland Trade Center #3
7501 Greenway Center Dr, Suite 760
Greenbelt MD 20770
Tel: 301-313-0855
Fax: 301-313-0912
www.acaom.org

American Association of Acupuncture and Oriental Medicine
PO Box 162340
Sacramento CA 95816
Tel: 866-455-7999
www.aaaomonline.org

National Certification Commission for Acupuncture and Oriental Medicine
76 South Laura St, Suite 1290
Jacksonville FL 32202
Tel: 904-598-1005

Fax: 904-598-5001
nccaom.org

The Association of Traditional Chinese Medicine (UK)
5A Grosvenor House
1 High Street
Edgware
London, England
HA8 7TA
Tel: 020 8951 3030
Fax: 020 8951 3030
www.atcm.co.uk

Australian Acupuncture and Chinese Medicine Association
PO Box 1635
Cooparoo DC QLD 4151
Tel: 61 (0)7 3324 2599
Fax: 61 (0)7 3394 2399
www.acupuncture.org.au

Federation of Acupuncture and Oriental Medicine Regulatory
Agencies
Pete Gonzalez, President
Arizona State Acupuncture Board of Examiners
1400 W. Washington, Suite 230
Phoenix AZ 85007
Tel: 602-364-0145
www.faomra.com

The World Federation of Acupuncture–Moxibustion Societies
www.wfas.org.cn/en/

The World Health Organization
www.who.int/en/

Websites of Interest

www.xiaolanhealthcentre.com

www.chinesehealing.com

tcm.health-info.org

www.acupuncturetoday.com

acupuncture.com

www.aworldofacupuncture.com

www.sacredlotus.com

www.rootdown.us

www.acupuncturetoday.com

www.chinesemedicinetools.com

chinesemedicinedatabase.com

www.tcmassistant.com

www.nccam.nih.gov

www.aobta.org

www.acupunctureresearch.org

INDEX

DR. XIAOLAN ZHAO was working as a Western-trained surgeon in China when she became interested in Traditional Chinese Medicine (TCM) and decided to go back to school to earn a degree in TCM. After immigrating to Canada in the late 1980s, she opened a TCM clinic in Toronto. Since then, her practice has grown to more than 12,000 devoted patients.